Understand Alzheimer's

Understand Alzheimer's

A First-Time Caregiver's Plan to Understand & Prepare for Alzheimer's & Dementia

CALISTOGA PRESS

For general information on our other products and services or to obtain technical support, please contact our Customer Care Department within the United States at (866) 744-2665, or outside the United States at (510) 253-0500.

Calistoga Press publishes its books in a variety of electronic and print formats. Some content that appears in print may not be available in electronic books, and vice versa.

TRADEMARKS: Calistoga Press and the Calistoga Press logo are trademarks or registered trademarks of Callisto Media Inc. and/or its affiliates, in the United States and other countries, and may not be used without written permission. All other trademarks are the property of their respective owners. Calistoga Press is not associated with any product or vendor mentioned in this book.

ISBN: Print 978-1-62315-300-7 | eBook 978-1-62315-301-4

Contents

Introduction

While you may not know much about Alzheimer's disease, you most likely do know someone in your life—a relative, a friend, or a neighbor—who has been diagnosed. You have heard how this devastating, elusive disease changes people and their families irrevocably—altering behavior, reducing normal functioning, and robbing people of cherished memories.

If you are reading this book, you are probably grappling with a recent diagnosis of someone close to you and wondering how you can best support that person, now and as the disease progresses. You may even be considering becoming that person's primary caregiver. But what does being a primary caregiver actually mean and require? Are you the best-equipped person to care for your loved one, and if so, what do you need to know to manage the care of the patient, as well as yourself? As you search for answers and validation, you also may be searching for a clear understanding of what an Alzheimer's diagnosis means both medically and emotionally. Finally, you may be unsure whether the important role of caregiver is the best option for you or your loved one and need a resource to help you weigh options and provide facts necessary to help you commit to this life choice.

This book endeavors to supply the facts and separate them from the myths you may have heard about the disease, and to give you useful, step-by-step, up-to-date information throughout each of the progressive stages of Alzheimer's disease. This information will help you make the decision about the level of participation in caregiving that will match your abilities, your loved one's financial situation, and the realities of your own life and commitments.

Caregivers take many roles and come from many different relationships with the person who needs care. Instead of becoming a primary caregiver—making a round-the-clock, live-in commitment to your loved one—you can make certain that the person with Alzheimer's lives in a safe environment, receives the assistance he needs with activities of daily living, and has an appropriate level of supervision without taking care of all of his needs yourself. Your loved one may not need round-the-clock supervision until the disease reaches its severe stage, making it possible for you to serve as a part-time caregiver for a few hours a day. Perhaps the person only needs help with managing finances, mail, and transportation, allowing you to provide these services on an as-needed basis.

You may find that you are able to share the caregiving responsibility with other family members: siblings, children, grandchildren, or nieces and nephews. Even if you are unable to directly support your loved one, you may still be instrumental in providing support to the primary caregiver(s). The more information you have about Alzheimer's disease and its progression, the more genuinely helpful you can be to your family members.

It's also possible that your loved one with Alzheimer's has the financial means to allow you to hire support from a home health agency or to relocate the person to one of the many excellent assisted-living facilities that provide memory care. If so, while you will not need to provide the primary care yourself, your role in supervising your loved one's care in such a living situation is just as instrumental to the person's quality of life. It will be up to you and your family to provide outings, visits, shopping, financial management, and other services as your loved one loses the ability to perform these tasks. You will also need to be vigilant, making certain that the facility you've chosen provides the high-quality, compassionate care your loved one needs and deserves.

While this book is a guide to understanding the caregiving role in general, many of the chapters are directed toward the role of the primary caregiver. If you decide to take on this role, you will face elements of the caregiver job that task you physically, mentally, emotionally, and spiritually—but you may also be embarking on one of the most rewarding experiences of your life.

Caution: Life Changes Ahead

When you become the caregiver for a person with Alzheimer's, you can expect your life to mold itself around the daily routine and needs of that person, not the other way around. You are likely to take on tasks you never imagined yourself doing with adults, especially if they were once caregivers to you. You will need to keep them safe in their own home and eventually assume more responsibility of their daily needs such as assisting with bathing, dressing, and personal hygiene—a role reversal that you may find challenging on many levels. You may find your sleep interrupted and your paid work difficult to complete. You may have no idea what will come next as control over your well-ordered life transfers to forces outside yourself.

This guide will help you navigate the twists and turns of Alzheimer's disease, from the minor forgetfulness that marks its early stages to the dramatic effects of the late-stage illness. Becoming familiar with the symptoms and behaviors of Alzheimer's will help make the advancement of the disease more predictable, and will help you prepare your home, your loved one, and yourself for the situation that comes next. Each chapter addresses a specific aspect of the disease and the way it may affect your caregiving role.

You have already shown tremendous initiative and compassion by considering or accepting the role of caregiver. This book will help you be the best you can be in your new endeavor while providing optimal care to your loved one.

One last note: though more women than men are diagnosed with Alzheimer's disease, the use of "she" in this book when referring to a caretaker or to someone affected with Alzheimer's does not indicate that the same information is not also true for a man, and vice versa with the use of "he."

You, Your Loved One, and Alzheimer's Disease

CHAPTER ONE

Understanding the Diagnosis

As frightening as a diagnosis of Alzheimer's may be, it may help you to know that you and your loved one are far from alone. The Alzheimer's Association tells us that 5.2 million Americans had this disease in 2013, and all but 200,000 of them were age 65 and older at the time of diagnosis. With the Baby Boomer generation reaching retirement age, the number of people with Alzheimer's is expected to increase—up to 7.1 million by 2025.

Before you can begin to determine how you and your loved one will approach the days ahead, it's important to have a full understanding of Alzheimer's and what this diagnosis means to you, your family, and your way of life.

What Is Alzheimer's Disease?

What you know of Alzheimer's disease today may be limited, but just about everyone knows this much: this progressive disease damages the brain, kills brain cells, wipes out memories, and changes the way an otherwise healthy, vital human being perceives and functions in the world.

Alzheimer's is the most common cause of dementia, a broad category of disorders that cause memory loss, reduction in basic intellectual skills, and a loss in the ability to communicate and connect with other people.

Everyone's brain contains billions of nerve cells, or neurons. These cells communicate with one another to form massive networks, transmitting signals to allow our bodies to move, think, feel, smell, see, and hear. When the messages between these neurons transmit properly—as they do for most of our lives—people function normally, take in new information, form memories, and enjoy a healthy life.

To keep information moving from one neuron to another, our brain cells work hard every second. They build communication networks among one another, take in oxygen and nutrients from the bloodstream, and dispose of waste once they've used the nutrients. Brain cells also store information in the form of memories and act as random processors, accessing these memories instantly as we need them.

Alzheimer's disease and other forms of dementia interfere with this healthy exchange of information and processing of supplies. While a number of kinds of dementia come from trauma to the brain—a stroke, a blow to the head, or other illnesses described later in this chapter—Alzheimer's disease causes a series of changes in the brain that are not present in other forms of dementia. Doctors can see these changes by using advanced brain scans.

Researchers at universities and laboratories around the world are working to understand how this disease begins and whether changes in the brain might reveal the root causes. Today we know that the brains of people with Alzheimer's disease have two important abnormalities that are not found in patients with other forms of dementia: plaques and tangles.

Protein deposits called plaques appear between nerve cells, spreading through the cerebral cortex—the outside layer of the brain. This part of the brain controls thinking, problem solving, sensations, and the formation of memories. Researchers believe that these plaques, made of a protein called beta-amyloid, interfere with these functions.

Tangles are knots of tau, another protein, that concentrate inside nerve cells. Think of these knots like the invasive plants in your yard, tangling around your shrubs and trees and inhibiting your desirable plants' ability to grow. Tangles cut off the flow of nutrients to the brain's neurons and keep the neurons from communicating with one another, eventually making it impossible for the brain to function properly.

Scientists do not yet understand where these Alzheimer's-specific plaques and tangles come from or what can be done to stop them from forming. Researchers do know that when neurons in the brain cannot get the nutrients they need to thrive and cannot communicate with one another, they die, and with them go short-term memories and learned behaviors stored within them.

Plaques and tangles do not show up on brain scans—in fact, doctors can't see them until there's an autopsy. That's why a diagnosis of Alzheimer's tends to come with a qualifying word: "possible Alzheimer's disease" or "probable Alzheimer's disease." Doctors judge the presence of Alzheimer's based on a combination of physical and mental symptoms that tend to be present in virtually all cases.

Today a diagnosis of Alzheimer's signals the approaching end of life. The Alzheimer's Association tells us that Alzheimer's disease is the fifth leading cause of death in people over sixty-five in the United States, that it afflicts women more than men, and that it is the only leading cause of death for which there is no prevention or cure. While many other causes of death (breast or prostate cancer, heart disease and stroke, and complications of HIV) are becoming preventable, Alzheimer's deaths have skyrocketed by 68 percent in the last decade.

The good news is that there has been more progress in research on Alzheimer's in the last fifteen years than at any other time in history. The more that scientists learn about this disease, the more treatments they can discover, and the closer they get to preventive measures that may slow the progress of Alzheimer's and related dementias.

Dementia Versus Alzheimer's

While all Alzheimer's causes dementia, not all dementia comes from Alzheimer's. Sixty to eighty percent of dementia cases are diagnosed as Alzheimer's disease, but other forms of dementia come from different kinds of damage to the brain.

Vascular dementia results from changes in blood vessels related to a large or small stroke. A stroke takes place when an obstruction in blood flow—called a thrombosis—forms in the brain and suffocates blood cells until they die. A ruptured artery also can cause a stroke, interrupting blood flow and starving the neurons to death.

In most cases, other symptoms besides a loss of cognitive function will appear, such as a lack of motor coordination, confusion, difficulty speaking, loss of sight, or difficulty performing basic tasks.

Clusters of a protein called alpha-synuclein appearing in the brain's cerebral cortex indicate the patient has a less common condition called dementia with Lewy bodies. This protein also appears in the brains of people with Parkinson's disease—another common cause of dementia—and people with either condition may eventually develop memory loss, changes in reasoning, and trouble understanding visual information. Those with Lewy body dementia have symptoms similar to those with Alzheimer's and other forms of dementia: changes in alertness from one time of day to another, hallucinations, delusions, balance problems, and rigid muscles.

In all of these forms of dementia, the disease or damage may be combined with the destructive abnormalities of Alzheimer's disease, making a single diagnosis inappropriate. When this happens, doctors call the condition mixed dementia—a term that family members of patients often consider inconclusive. For example, an 85-year-old woman who does not recognize her grandchildren (Alzheimer's) also may see people who are not there (Lewy bodies). The doctor will correctly diagnose mixed dementia in this case, opening the door to a wider variety of treatment options.

A number of much less common causes of dementia also may be at work in your loved one's case. Your doctor will have information on these rare conditions if one of them turns up in the examination.

Early Detection and Why It Matters

Early-Stage Warning Signs

If you are reading this book because you suspect that your loved one has Alzheimer's disease or related dementia, you may be seeing some or all of the ten warning signs that raise questions about your family member's mental health:

1. Memory loss that disrupts daily life

2. Challenges planning or solving problems

3. Difficulty completing familiar tasks

4. Confusion with time or place

5. Trouble understanding visual images or spatial relationships

6. New problems with language, including inability to find the word he wants to use, sustain a train of thought, and understand what is being said to him

7. Misplacing things and becoming unable to retrace steps

8. Decreased or poor judgment

9. Withdrawal from work or social activities

10. Changes in mood or personality

Early detection can be a key component in curbing the early symptoms of the disease, by connecting your loved one with treatments that can slow down the memory loss temporarily and improve his quality of life. The sooner treatment begins, the longer your loved one can live with a minimum of symptoms.

In addition, with so much focus on Alzheimer's throughout the worldwide scientific research community, clinical trials may be available to your family member that may not only help slow the disease's progression, but may help scientists understand the disease and speed their progress toward new treatments, or even a cure.

Alzheimer's is a complex disease that will require a number of changes in your loved one's life—and in yours as well. When you recognize the early symptoms and a diagnosis is given, you can begin to plan immediately for your loved one's care before the disease progresses. Equally important, your loved one can be involved in the care decisions, helping you plan while he has the cognitive ability to do so. This can alleviate a great deal of tension, hesitation, and guilt later on, when you will need to make decisions based on your own good judgment and your loved one's financial situation. (You'll find more on this subject in chapters 11 and 12.)

Finally, the sooner you know about your loved one's disease, the longer you have to explore all of the options available to you for his care. Having to make unexpected decisions at the last minute can mean that you must grab the first option you find for long-term care, short-term respite care, or another living option—which may lead to regrets and family conflict.

The Diagnosis

No one test conclusively proves that a patient has Alzheimer's disease or another dementia, but the combination of a number of tests and exams allows the primary care physician to make an initial diagnosis and a referral to a neurologist, who will narrow down the diagnosis.

- **Medical history.** Your doctor will ask about your loved one's physical health, including all of the medications he is taking and any illnesses he has, as both may cause symptoms of dementia. Something as common as a urinary tract infection can cause hallucinations and dementia, so it's important that you and your loved one supply all of the information requested.

  - Make a list of the symptoms that you, your family members or friends, and any caregivers to your loved one have noticed.

  - Take a list of your loved one's medications and dosages—both over the counter and prescription—or bring the bottles.

  - Bring a pad and pen to the appointment, and write down what the doctor tells you about test results and other examinations. It can be hard to remember exactly what the doctor said, especially if the news you receive is not what you hoped for.

- **Physical exam.** The doctor(s) will check your loved one's blood pressure, pulse, temperature, heart and lungs, and other baseline vital signs to get a clear picture of his health. Your doctor also will want to know about the patient's exercise regimen, diet, use of tobacco and alcohol, sleep schedule, and other basic activities of daily living. Expect the medical staff to order blood and urine tests.

- **Neurological exam.** Many of the things your primary care physician does during a regular physical are actually meant to test a patient's brain and nervous system to be sure they are in working order. Your doctor will check your loved one's reflexes, strength, eye movement, ability to feel and hear normally, and ability to speak.

- **Brain imaging.** When your primary care physician refers your loved one to a neurologist, he probably will have an MRI (magnetic resonance imaging) or a CT or CAT (computer tomography) scan, two critically important tests that help doctors rule out causes of dementia, such as stroke, that may mimic Alzheimer's disease.

- **Mental tests.** Simple tests can help medical professionals determine if your loved one's memory has been affected by disease. The testing clinician conducts a mini-mental state exam (MMSE) by asking the patient a series of basic questions, with a potential high score of 30 points on the exam. If the patient scores lower than 20 points, progressive dementia is indicated.

The doctor will also talk with the patient to check for signs of depression, one of several mood disorders that can cause memory loss and other dementia symptoms.

Frequently Asked Questions About Alzheimer's Disease

You probably have many questions and concerns about Alzheimer's disease, but you might not know what to ask first. The following are a few of the questions many people have when first confronted with the disease.

1. **Doesn't everyone get Alzheimer's as they get old?**

   We all will have some form of memory loss as we get older, but for most of us, it's a much milder kind of loss—for example, opening the refrigerator and forgetting what we wanted inside, or misplacing our keys. A memory has formed and momentarily becomes inaccessible, but it returns in a few minutes. For people with Alzheimer's disease, brain cells are damaged and die, and this erases some memories altogether.

2. **Can younger people get Alzheimer's?**

   It's much less common, but early onset Alzheimer's afflicts people as young as their 30s. About three percent of the people who have Alzheimer's today are younger than 65.

3. **Is there anything my family should not do to avoid getting Alzheimer's?**

   So far, the various claims that certain substances cause Alzheimer's disease have not held up under scientific investigation. Aluminum, once believed to cause Alzheimer's, has been proven to have no effect at all in the development of the disease. The U.S. Food and Drug Administration has ruled out the artificial sweetener aspartame as a cause of Alzheimer's, and the doctor who proposed that flu shots caused the disease has been discredited along with his theory—in fact, flu shots are now linked to a reduced risk of Alzheimer's.

4. **Will diet keep me from getting Alzheimer's?**

   While maintaining a healthy diet, getting regular exercise, and focusing on overall good health are always advisable goals for a long life, there is no "super food" that will prevent Alzheimer's disease. Your best bet is the same kind of diet that will help you avoid heart disease and diabetes: low saturated fat, low cholesterol, and a balance of protein, starch, fruits, and vegetables. A long-term study has shown that people who are obese in middle age have twice the risk of developing dementia later in life—and those with high cholesterol and high blood pressure have six times the risk! A heart-healthy diet also increases your natural intake of important vitamins like vitamin E, C, B-12, and folate, all of which may be important in lowering your risk of Alzheimer's disease.

5. **Will staying mentally active and doing puzzles keep me from getting Alzheimer's?**

   Puzzles, brainteasers, games, and reading regularly can help strengthen your brain by creating new brain cells and keeping the connections active between neurons. While there is no single research study that concludes that crossword or jigsaw puzzles actually prevent Alzheimer's disease, maintaining your curiosity and stimulating your brain may simply keep it more fit, potentially reducing the risk of dementia later in life.

6. Are there medications that will stop Alzheimer's disease from getting worse?

So far, the available medications will slow the progress of the disease for up to a year at best. There are no medications that will stop the disease indefinitely, or that will cure it.

7. My parent has Alzheimer's disease. Should I get genetic testing?

Research does show that you have a greater risk of getting Alzheimer's disease if others in your family have it, but there are no guarantees. In October 2013, the International Genomics of Alzheimer's Project—the first global collaborative effort to discover and map the genes that contribute to Alzheimer's—announced the identification of eleven genes linked to Alzheimer's, based on a study of more than seventy-four thousand patients in fifteen countries. Before this study, four gene mutations had been identified: three are linked to early onset Alzheimer's (You will find more on the stages of Alzheimer's in chapter 6), while the fourth (known as APOE-e4) increases the likelihood of developing the late-onset disease—though it is by no means certain that you will get Alzheimer's even if you have the gene. If you feel that genetic testing is important to you, discuss it with your doctor before you make the decision. You may hope for the peace of mind that comes with a negative finding, but if you discover that you have the mutated gene, it might lead to a lifetime of anxiety while you wait for symptoms to appear.

8. What about stem cell treatment?

The use of stem cells to change the course of Alzheimer's disease has challenges that are not found when used in parts of the body other than the brain. The disease affects many kinds of brain cells rather than just one kind, and scientists do not yet know if all of these different cells can be duplicated by stem cells. In addition, healthy brain cells created from stem cells will face the same aggressive issues the original cells faced—plaques and tangles that contaminate healthy brain cells. Research continues, but there are no cures just around the corner.

9. How long will my loved one live with Alzheimer's?

Patients with Alzheimer's disease live anywhere from two to twenty years after their diagnosis. The average life expectancy is eight to ten years. The Alzheimer's Foundation of America says that most people with this disease develop another illness, and the majority die of pneumonia rather than of Alzheimer's.

....

In October 2013, the International Genomics of Alzheimer's Project announced the identification of eleven genes linked to Alzheimer's.

....

CHAPTER TWO

Choosing to Become a Caregiver

Your first impulse when your spouse, parent, or sibling receives the diagnosis of Alzheimer's disease may be to become the primary caregiver for your loved one. Perhaps you have known other family caregivers in your lifetime, or you simply feel that being the primary caregiver would be the best situation for your loved one and for you. Allowing the person to continue to live at home or move into your home for as long as possible may feel like a far more preferable solution to you than moving him into a residential facility, even if it's the best assisted-living center or memory-care unit of a local senior living community, especially in the earlier stages of the disease. This book will help you decide what living and caregiving situation is best for both you and your loved one.

If you choose to become a caregiver, you join a long history of extended families caring for their own in the comfort and loving atmosphere of their own homes. It's a position that will require vigilance to keep your loved one safe, sacrifice of a great deal of your personal time, and some significant changes in your relationship with the person to whom you will give your care. Chances are you do not have medical or patient aide training for this responsibility—and if you do, you have an even better idea of what will be involved.

If the caregiving role is entirely new to you, here are some issues you need to consider before making the commitment to take on this challenge.

Coping with the Diagnosis

You and the patient will have an emotional response to the diagnosis of Alzheimer's disease, and those emotions may become more pronounced for both of you over time.

Your loved one faces losing his independence, perhaps one of the hardest life changes that anyone can face. No longer able to live on his own, to work, to drive a car, or to accomplish the same tasks he may have throughout his working life, your loved one may become frustrated, angry, and depressed. Anxiety often comes with the inability to do simple things, especially if your loved one fears being embarrassed in a social situation if he becomes confused or can't form the words he wants to say. This leads to alienation from friends and family, which leads to loneliness and more depression.

All of these early responses to the diagnosis are normal, but they can be very disturbing, and they can reduce your loved one's quality of life just as his disease is separating him from all of the things he enjoys: friends, hobbies, family, work, and the freedom to do as he pleases. The emotional reactions can also complicate your early days as the caregiver, especially if this role signals a major change in your relationship—for example, if you will be caring for a parent who has spent much of his life looking after you.

Just as your family member faces many changes in his life that may create lowered feelings and bitterness, you also face a major change. As you become the caregiver, you may feel that you need to sweep all of your feelings under the rug while you do your best to help your loved one. This is neither healthy nor advisable, as it will only create feelings of anger and resentment. This is a journey you and your loved one will take together, so share the exploration by learning all you can together about Alzheimer's disease and its implications for both of your lives.

Is Caregiving Right for You?

The fact is, caregiving is not for everyone. Before you make the commitment to care for your loved one at home, consider these questions about the kinds of responsibilities you may have to take on.

1. **Do you have the time and the skills to perform tasks including cooking, cleaning, running errands, providing transportation, and managing finances?**

    Chances are that you do these things for yourself already, but if your loved one with Alzheimer's disease is not living with you, you will find yourself the housekeeper for two residences.

2. **Are you the primary caregiver for young children?**

    You may want desperately to take care of your loved one, but consider whether doing so would take away the attention necessary to raise a young family. If you feel moving your loved one into your home is an option, discuss safety issues that may affect small children with family members and physicians.

3. **How do you feel about providing personal care—bathing, dressing, or eventually feeding your loved one?**

    These needs may change the dynamic of your relationship, and if so, do you feel you can develop a comfort level with these tasks?

4. **Do you have the authority to make decisions for your loved one? In other words, do you have durable power of attorney, so that you can make health care and financial decisions when necessary?**

    If not, who in your family can take on this responsibility, and do you have a cooperative relationship with that person?

5. **Do you know your own limits?**

    At some point, you are likely to need outside assistance to handle health or behavior issues with your loved one. Knowing when you have reached the end of your skill set—or your endurance—and bringing in outside help can turn a potentially hazardous situation into a safe one.

6. **Do you have a job that permits the responsibilities of caregiving?**

If you continue to work while you have primary responsibility for your loved one, there may be times when you need to break away from work at a moment's notice to deal with a difficult situation at home. If your career does not permit this, you may need to look at other caregiving options or change your work situation.

7. **How is your own health—both physical and mental?**

Becoming a caregiver can be taxing to your physical strength, and it can require long hours and double-duty between two households—not to mention the potential for lost sleep, sadness, and all kinds of unexpected feelings about your caregiving situation.

8. **What kind of support network can you put in place?**

Taking over the care of your loved one does not mean that the rest of your family is off the hook. You will need days off, help with large tasks, participation in making family decisions, and people who will listen when you need to talk. If you don't have family, or if your family members are too far away geographically to be part of the picture, then you will need to enlist the help of community services in your area. (You will find more about how to find this help in chapter 11.)

9. **What is your financial situation?**

Can you leave your job when your caregiving responsibilities increase? If your loved one has financial resources, it may make sense that you are paid for the work you are doing as caregiver. If you truly cannot afford to take time away from work for an indefinite period and there are no other resources to draw upon to support your caregiving role, you may not be the right person to take on this responsibility.

....

In 2012, 15.4 million caregivers provided more than 17.5 billion hours of unpaid care for Alzheimer's patients, valued at $216 billion.

....

Educate Yourself

The first step in becoming a caregiver is to learn all you can about what the responsibility will entail. Becoming informed will not only give you the information you need to understand the skills involved but also help you determine if you are the right person to take on the caregiving role.

Many of the behaviors that you will encounter as a caregiver to someone afflicted with Alzheimer's disease are very specific to dementia patients. You many find it very helpful to take a course in caregiving for dementia, where you can see and hear an instructor demonstrate the best way to handle behaviors and also learn techniques to redirect a patient or to interrupt a cycle of behavior.

Your local chapter of the Alzheimer's Association can help you find courses for caregivers. If there is no chapter in your area, inquire with senior-living communities that specialize in dementia, or check with your local community college to see if you can take a caregiving course. This may mean that you need to attend a course during one or two evenings a week, so alert your support network that you will need someone to step in for you so you can receive this training.

Transitioning into Your New Role

You may discover that you already have been a caregiver to your loved one for some time, but that you did not identify yourself as one. Before your family member received the diagnosis of Alzheimer's disease, you knew that things had started to change in his life. You had taken over the cleaning of his house or took meals to him every few days. Perhaps you had been keeping your loved one's financial records up to date, paying the bills, and tracking his checking account online. You may already be mowing the lawn, raking leaves, or shoveling your loved one's front walk. All of these things are part of the caregiver's role.

Even as you become the full-time caregiver for your loved one, you still may feel that you're just keeping an eye on things. Caregiving at first may be as simple as driving your loved one to medical appointments and taking over his medication management—making sure he takes his pills at the right times. If your loved one is in the early stage of dementia, he may not yet have issues that require round-the-clock supervision. This is a good time to learn all you can about what is to come, before a sudden change in your family member's behavior forces you into an emergency situation.

....

Nearly 15 percent of caregivers for people with Alzheimer's or another dementia are long-distance caregivers.

....

Relationship Changes

Over time, you will experience a larger transition. You will need to assist your loved one with activities of daily living: bathing, dressing, eating, and going to the bathroom (what the eldercare profession calls "toileting"). At this point, you will feel more like a caregiver, but you may find the change to this stage particularly hard to make. It represents a major shift in your relationship with the person in your care, whether he or she is your parent, spouse, sibling, aunt, or uncle.

A study conducted at the University of Pittsburgh School of Medicine discovered that the transition to helping the relative with activities of daily living has the most pronounced effect on the caregiver, both because of the physical exertion involved and because of the emotional factors in seeing a loved one lose the ability to do these things for himself. As if to make things tougher, your family member may feel minimized in his role and may react negatively to your new position in his life.

If you are caring for your spouse, you may take on responsibilities that have always been your spouse's contribution to your relationship: handling financial matters, doing chores that he or she always did, doing your annual taxes, or repairing items around the house. You may need to make major decisions alone that you used to make together. This can make you second-guess your own judgment, or feel overwhelmed or fearful.

Perhaps most challenging of all in becoming a caregiver to your spouse is the potential loss of intimacy, conversation, and affection that you have enjoyed throughout your years together. Alzheimer's and accompanying depression may change your spouse's interest in sex, and some medications may reduce sex drive or potency even more. At the same time, your own interest in intimacy may be lessened because of the changes you see in your spouse, as well as the energy you expend every day in his or her care. None of these changes are anyone's fault. Look for other ways to maintain that familiar connection between you, even if sex is out of the question.

Preparing for Caregiving

Use this checklist to help you prepare your home and yourself for your caregiving role.

✓   Pharmacy location and phone number (is there a drive-through/will they deliver?)

✓   List of medications, dosages, and times they should be given

✓   Calendar for medical appointments

✓   Contact numbers of doctor, hospital, people you can call in an emergency

✓   Health insurance policy

✓   Adult day care address and phone number (see chapter 11)

✓   Personal emergency response system, like LifeAlert, for your loved one to use if they fall or need help when you are not available

✓   Remove any obstacles or slipping hazards such as throw rugs, mats, and obstructions on staircases or near doors

✓   Bring all financial and legal documents together in one place (see chapter 12)

....

Caregiving can be an isolating experience, but nothing in the job description requires you to do it alone.

....

Essential Steps to Getting Started as a Caregiver

Choosing to become a caregiver is a very difficult step that typically involves a lot of emotions. Following these ten steps will help ensure a successful start to your new role as caregiver.

1. **Make a family decision.** Get together with your siblings, spouse, children, and any other family members who should be involved in your loved one's care. If your family is far-flung across the country, use Skype (or whichever app you like) to involve them in the family meeting. Talk through everything you have observed and your loved one's diagnosis, and determine the next steps you need to take as a family. Even if your family members have issues with one another, it's important to involve everyone you can to achieve at least a majority vote with all family members, if not a consensus. This is the time for all family members to voice their opinions about what's best for the person with Alzheimer's, and it's good to know from the beginning if family conflicts are likely to arise.

2. **Gather information.** The more you know about Alzheimer's disease and the changes that will take place over time, the better you can plan for what's ahead.

3. **Get a professional assessment.** Your loved one's doctor, your local hospital, an eldercare organization, or a home health-care organization can recommend a case manager or home-care professional to make a formal assessment of your loved one's current needs and what they are likely to be in the future. This is an established, state-regulated process that will be invaluable in planning your next steps. (See chapter 11 for more information.)

4. **Determine what your loved one can afford.** Most people are not independently wealthy, but your family member may have the means available (or may be entitled to benefits if he or she is a veteran) to pay for professional in-home assistance a few times a week, or even for several years in an assisted-living situation. Gather all of his financial information—bank accounts, credit cards, annuities,

investments, home appraisal, and (if you're lucky) long-term care insurance—so you and your family can make an educated decision based on all of the means available. (See chapter 12 for more information.)

5. **Determine who in your family has power of attorney.** Chances are that your loved one chose someone to whom he gave *durable power of attorney*, making that person the attorney-in-fact who can make legal, financial, and health care decisions when your loved one can no longer make those decisions for himself. To activate the power of attorney, that person must have the original, signed, notarized document. (Once your loved one has been diagnosed with advanced- or late-stage Alzheimer's disease, he cannot legally sign any document. If there is no power of attorney, someone in your family will need to be appointed by a court. Chapter 12 discusses this process and information on durable power of attorney in further detail.)

6. **Collect all legal documents.** In addition to the power of attorney, your loved one may have executed a health care proxy and/or a living will, stating his wishes for end-of-life medical care. Other documents you will need are listed in chapter 12.

7. **Plan for safe, comprehensive care.** Put together a plan that covers all of the things your loved one will need, from help with activities of daily living to medical requirements. This plan will change as your loved one's needs change, but it will help you look ahead to the things you will need down the road as well as the steps you must take now.

8. **Determine your support network.** Who are the relatives that you can call on for assistance at a moment's notice? Which of your friends will stay in touch with you, even if they feel discomfort around your disabled loved one? These people and others—a support group, a home health care service, and the local chapter of the Alzheimer's Association or another eldercare organization—become your network of support. Caregiving can be an isolating experience, but nothing in the job description requires you to do it alone.

9. **Make your home safe.** That little throw rug in your kitchen may look adorable against the tile floor, but it's a tripping hazard—as are any obstacles on your stairs or near doorways. Reduce the potential for falls and a number of other accidents that become possible as Alzheimer's progresses. See the checklist in chapter 5 to help you.

10. **Establish some time for yourself.** Chapter 3 is devoted entirely to this important step, but the sooner you build some personal time into your schedule, the more likely it is that you will take that time.

CHAPTER THREE

Taking Care of Yourself

You will hear this refrain from friends and relatives in almost every conversation you have with them about your loved one's care: "Remember, you have to take care of yourself, too!"

Rarely is this advice followed by any helpful hints about *how* to do this. A patient with Alzheimer's often requires round-the-clock care, especially as the disease progresses and your loved one develops new, more pronounced symptoms, like switching day for night (sleeping by day and wandering the house at night), general wandering, and obsessive behaviors.

It's not uncommon for caregivers to deal with fatigue, sadness, guilt, anger, and overall stress, and at the same time to feel as if they cannot take time away or do not deserve rest or respite, much less any activity they might enjoy. This conflicting set of physical issues and emotions can make it more and more difficult to function effectively as a caregiver. Over time, stress and exhaustion wear down the caregiver, potentially creating a new set of issues.

Research shows that caregivers suffer from increased rates of physical problems, including acid reflux, headaches, and aching joints or muscles, and an increased tendency to develop serious illnesses. Obesity also becomes an issue for caregivers who give up a healthy diet and regular exercise while they care for their loved ones.

It will never be easy, but you can reduce the risk of developing physical and mental health issues by addressing the need to take care of yourself from the beginning of your caregiving relationship.

Practice Self-Compassion

First, stop beating yourself up. Alzheimer's disease is a progressive illness, one that even the most comprehensive expert care cannot cure or curtail. As the caregiver, you can manage the symptoms and look out for your loved one's safety, but you cannot keep them from getting worse. What is happening to your loved one is not your fault, his fault, or anyone's fault.

When you are in the throes of dealing with your family member and the disease, it can be easy to slip into anger, guilt, and regret over the changes in your loved one's personality and behavior. This self-critical reaction—the search for accountability and determination of who's responsible, and the inevitable decision that it's you—is the path that you've probably been taught since grade school: find what's wrong with you and fix it, and you will achieve success.

Has that worked for you? Chances are it hasn't, and studies have shown that this kind of self-criticism only undermines your self-esteem, leading to exactly the opposite effect from the one you were hoping to achieve. Instead, Kristin Neff, PhD, a researcher at the University of Texas at Austin, recommends that you treat yourself the way you would treat a sibling or friend who faced the same situation that you're experiencing now: drop the self-criticism and practice self-compassion.

Dr. Neff suggests that you be kind and understanding with yourself, and realize that the struggle you're going through makes you feel alone and isolated, as if you're the only one in the world who has ever had these feelings or made a mistake. Note the language you use when you chastise yourself. Would you say such things to another person? If you are being harder on yourself than you would ever be on someone else, it's time to refocus and change the words you use to describe yourself.

Guided meditation, prayer, or just taking a break to go outside and breathe can be helpful in restoring equanimity when you catch yourself being self-critical. Even if you can only spare a few minutes, the practice of breathing deeply, focusing your mind on a single thought, and repeating a self-affirming phrase can break a vicious cycle of self-loathing and doubt.

Self-compassion is not selfish or self-indulgent, Dr. Neff concludes. You are simply redirecting your thoughts and criticism in a way that helps you past the most difficult moments and halts the avalanche of recrimination you heap onto yourself. You are suffering, just as your loved one is. You have the right and the need to alleviate this suffering.

Maintain Balance

Issues and emergencies arise without warning, but for the most part, a caregiver can establish a routine that keeps home tasks, work life, and some recreation or respite as part of the picture. Planning ahead, maintaining a schedule, and involving others can help you balance your work, your caregiving, and your personal needs.

- **Find an adult day program.** Senior centers often have programs for Alzheimer's patients, where they can interact with one another, enjoy recreational activities, have a hot lunch and snacks, or just sit in the company of others. Your loved one may be able to attend these programs five days a week or fewer as you prefer (and as he is able), giving you the peace of mind that he is in a safe place with others while you are at work or are taking a respite during the day.

....

A good adult day program seeks to enrich the lives of its participants through social activities. Look for a program that offers arts and crafts, games that stimulate the mind, chair exercises or other gentle movement, discussion groups, sing-alongs, and even some outings to local restaurants or events. Some programs include interaction with children, and some bring in therapy dogs or other animals.

....

- **Plan ahead.** Doctor appointments, physical and occupational therapy, visits by a home-health professional, and other activities can be scheduled in advance so you'll know to plan around them. Likewise, you can schedule your own pursuits into the mix—your evening class, your book-club meeting, or social time with friends—and ask your family members to spend some time with your loved one while you do these things.

- **Use digital communication.** Create a family email distribution list, and send updates to the entire family at once when you have something to tell them or need their assistance. It will be much easier to ask for help if they know that your loved one's disease is progressing, or if they are aware of changes you've observed or incidents that have happened. The more information they have, the more they can help you when you need them.

- **Be realistic about your commitment.** If you need to support yourself financially, there is only so much you can do during the workday to look after your loved one. If your loved one is calling you at work every day with a different (or the same) request or need, it's time to enlist the help of others.

- **Eat, sleep, exercise.** The only way you can continue to provide good care to your loved one is to stay healthy yourself. Share these activities with your loved one: cook and eat meals together, take a walk outside or through the mall, and maintain a sleep schedule for as long as the disease allows. When he no longer sleeps through the night, it's time to look at other care options: an overnight home health professional can let you get a good night's sleep while keeping your loved one from wandering in the middle of the night.

All of these points require one thing: asking for help from others.

Ask for Help

Why is this so difficult for caregivers to do? The answer can be complicated.

- Perhaps you feel that you made the commitment to take care of your family member, so caretaking should be your responsibility alone.

- Maybe you feel that others do not understand your loved one's affliction and that they will not care for them or be patient with them the way you are.

- You may be a person who does not like to ask for help as a general rule, feeling instead that you should be able to tackle any challenge or responsibility on your own.

- It could be that you don't want others judging the job you're doing, so you'd prefer they just stayed out of the situation.

- Longstanding family conflicts can keep people from asking their siblings or other family members for the help they need.

- Maybe you are feeling overwhelmed and you don't want others to suggest that it's time to start making other arrangements for your loved one.

- Or perhaps it's all of these reasons, and a few more that spring from your singular situation.

....

According to *Psychology Today*, as many as one-third of adult siblings describe their relationship as "rivalrous" or "distant." Well into adulthood and throughout their lives, siblings can be competitive, repeat the same arguments they started as children, and speak hurtfully to one another, essentially reducing themselves to squabbling like kids in a matter of minutes. When siblings start arguing about the care of a parent with Alzheimer's, all of these old hot buttons come to the surface once again.

....

Whatever the reasons, it's important to understand that asking for help is not optional. At some point in caring for someone with Alzheimer's disease, the job will become too large to do on your own. Later in this book, you'll find information on changing sleep patterns (sleeping by day and roaming the house at night), wandering, hallucinations, shadowing, verbal outbursts, and aggression, all symptoms of advancing illness that require twenty-four-hour, seven-day-a-week care—a level of care that no human being can do alone.

Even while your loved one has lost most of his cognitive abilities, you will need to leave the house without him on occasion, so someone else will need to be there with him while you are gone. It is unreasonable for you or your family to assume that you will never leave your loved one's side during this illness.

There's a flip side to this as well: your family members may be waiting for an opportunity to help, but they don't want to appear to interfere with your routine or seem as though they are second-guessing your skill or methods. Giving them an opportunity to help you may be just the opening they need to become more involved, providing you with a break when you need it.

When you know that you will need help, call one of your family members. Do this without attaching judgment to your words: For example, don't say, "You haven't done anything for us, so I hope you'll do this." Instead, ask for what you need in a factual manner: "I have a class on Thursday evenings, and I need someone to be with Dad while I go. Would you like to come over and visit with him on Thursdays?" You may be pleasantly surprised by the response.

At the same time, take a step back and think about how often your family members have offered you their help. Have you taken them up on these offers? The more you include them in the care of your loved one, the more likely they will be to see the responsibility for his care as a shared one, rather than your sole function. Remain open to offers of help, and keep a list of things that you could suggest that people do for you and your loved one. Running errands, staying with your loved one while you run errands, attending medical appointments, or spending a couple of hours with him on a weekend afternoon can be just the small gestures you need to feel refreshed and less stressed—and less alone.

....

Between 40 and 70 percent of caregivers have clinically significant symptoms of depression, worsening as the health of the person receiving care declines.

....

How to Manage Emotions

Anger, guilt, sadness, and anxiety are all likely to surface as you go forward as a caregiver. Your new role signals a number of changes in your life, from the amount of contact you have with your extended family to the disruption in your household if your loved one moves in with you. You know that this caregiving role will end one day, but you have no way to tell when that day may come. While caregiving can be rewarding as you form a special bond with your loved one, you also will face frustration, fear, self-doubt, and many other emotions you had not anticipated.

The statistics paint a fairly bleak picture. The Family Caregiver Alliance (FCA) states that between 40 and 70 percent of caregivers have clinically significant symptoms of depression, worsening as the health of the person receiving care declines. In caregivers for people with dementia, 30 to 40 percent suffer from a diagnosed clinical depression, as well as emotional stress. This does not necessarily improve when the person they cared for moves to a skilled nursing facility—in fact, many caregivers maintain their stress level and depression after this transition. Anxiety disorders like racing thoughts, phobias, shortness of breath, panic attacks, dizziness, and others can be common as well.

The FCA's research reveals a number of other mental-health issues in caregivers: high stress levels, anger, guilt, helplessness, frustration with the patient's lack of progress or continued decline, lowered self-esteem, worry, and a loss of self-identity. All of these issues tend to be more pronounced in female caregivers than in males—especially if the female caregiver is providing more than 36 hours of care per week.

What does this mean for you? Managing your own emotions can be a daunting task, especially when you are providing care for someone with Alzheimer's disease. The loved one with this illness may be unable to participate in finding solutions or in changing what may have become a bad situation—in fact, even if you try to talk it through with your loved one, he or she may not remember the conversation minutes later. This does little to relieve your frustration and helplessness.

It's important that you recognize the signs of anxiety disorders and depression in yourself and that your primary care doctor becomes aware of your caregiving situation, so he or she can help you monitor your symptoms and get the assistance you need.

- **Relaxation techniques** like meditation and yoga help some people relieve stress and anxiety.

- **Exercise** raises your endorphin levels, increasing your sense of well-being while it helps you channel negative emotions into physical energy. Even twenty minutes on a treadmill or a brisk walk can help to take the edge off frayed emotions.

- **Get respite.** Many assisted-living facilities offer short-term respite stays for people with Alzheimer's disease and other conditions, specifically to give caregivers a much-needed break from the stress of their responsibilities. Don't be afraid to arrange this kind of short-term solution for yourself; this is exactly what these senior living centers want to do for you.

- **Phone a friend.** Sometimes talking with a friend who understands your situation—or perhaps has been through it as well—can drain away the anger and frustration.

- **Tell your family.** Alerting your family to the stress levels you feel does not mean that you are weak. It does mean that you are self-aware enough to know your own limits. Involve your family in coming up with alternatives that will alleviate some of the stress, protecting your mental and physical health while making the best possible arrangement for your loved one.

- **Talk to your doctor.** Depression and anxiety disorders are chemical imbalances in your system, and they may need to be addressed with medications. The Centers for Disease Control tells us that 11 percent of Americans over age twelve were taking antidepressants in 2011, with women two and a half times more likely to take them than men. Additionally, the use of these drugs has become so widespread not only because of the availability of medications that make a positive difference in people's lives but also because the stigma associated with mental illness has decreased dramatically. If you have never taken antidepressants or antianxiety medication, discuss the pros and cons with your doctor.

Guilt

So here you are, taking on the primary responsibility of caring for your loved one, an act that proves your selflessness and your love for your family member. Somehow, though, you find yourself feeling guilty a great deal of the time, as if you're dropping the ball and not doing your best to address your loved one's physical health and well-being. What on earth is this about?

According to Maud Purcell, LCSW, in her essay "Guilt" for PsychCentral.com, you feel guilty when you believe that you have violated your own moral code of ethics. Perhaps you think that if you had intervened in your loved one's health earlier than you did, he would not have Alzheimer's disease today. You may believe that taking any kind of time for yourself is selfish, because your loved one continues to be confused and agitated. Or perhaps you snapped at your family member in anger, and now you feel that you've behaved horribly because he could not help his own actions.

You work through your feelings of guilt in your own way, and some of them seem never to disappear—but it *is* possible to forgive yourself for small infractions and change your own behavior, which will help you to avoid larger ones in the future. Look for the root cause of your guilt. In what way do you feel that you let yourself down? How can you recognize the potential for this action next time, and avoid taking the same action?

You can't change the things you did in the past, but you can go forward with stronger awareness, understand what you learned from the experience, and do better next time.

Taking Care of You:
Tips for Taking Care of Yourself

✓ Eat a balanced diet of healthy foods.

✓ Get regular exercise: 30 minutes a day, at least four days per week.

✓ Get the sleep you need to feel refreshed. The National Sleep Foundation says that the amount of sleep a person needs depends on the individual, but, as you are probably aware, studies suggest that seven to eight hours per night are required on average.

- ✓ Keep a schedule, and plan ahead for appointments, therapy, classes, and other activities.

- ✓ Enlist the help of friends and family whenever you can.

- ✓ Delegate tasks you don't have time to do: hire a cleaning service, have groceries delivered, and ask family members to provide transportation to appointments.

- ✓ Practice self-compassion instead of self-doubt.

- ✓ Use outside services to provide yourself with regular respite from caregiving.

- ✓ Learn from perceived mistakes, and forgive yourself for them.

- ✓ Know your limits, and be willing to make changes when you've reached them.

PART TWO

Stages, Symptoms, and Care

CHAPTER FOUR

Managing Health Care

As of this writing, the research community has not found a cure for Alzheimer's disease, or a way to prevent it. Managing your loved one's health care, then, will be geared toward maintaining quality of life for as long as possible while helping the patient function as normally as she can in daily activities.

Maintaining quality of life includes medication to temporarily improve memory, minimize mood swings, and reduce compulsive or repetitive behaviors. When your loved one can communicate with others and have a fairly cogent conversation, she can be more involved in social situations and enjoy visits with family members and friends—definitely a desirable outcome.

Your loved one's doctor will work with you to determine a treatment plan, including medications, physical therapy, and regular evaluations to monitor changes as they take place. Knowing what to expect will help you play an active role in this planning. Keep the doctor informed about the disease progression so that you and the doctor can adapt treatment as required.

....

Bring a pad and paper and make note of any instructions you receive about changes in your loved one's care.

....

Appointments

You or someone from your family should accompany your loved one on all appointments with the primary care physician and any specialists who are involved in the care. By definition, patients with Alzheimer's disease cannot be reliable in providing a medical history, discussing changes in their cognitive function or overall health, or remembering what doctors told them at the appointment. It may be helpful to you to keep an ongoing list of your questions for the doctor, and bring this list to the appointment to be sure you get the information you need. Bring a pad and paper and make note of the doctor's responses and of any instructions you receive about changes in your loved one's care.

The doctor should discuss with you the efficacy of the medications available for treatment of the symptoms of Alzheimer's disease. If your doctor prescribes one of these medications, be sure that you get information about possible side effects, reactions when combined with other medications, and the goals of using this medication. If the doctor tells you that a medication will slow the progression of the disease, ask him or her exactly what this means to help you set your own realistic expectations, as well as those of your loved one and other family members.

If you see your loved one's primary care physician regularly at these appointments, be aware that the doctor may ask questions about your own mental and physical health. The doctor is not asking these questions to imply that you are not doing your best to take care of your loved one. On the contrary, it's part of the doctor's responsibilities to be sure that the primary caregiver for the patient is faring well under the stress of the caregiving role. If the doctor makes recommendations to you or prescribes a medication to help you maintain your own good health, take these suggestions to heart. Doctors are trained to recognize the symptoms of stress and depression, two hazards of caregiving; if the doctor tells you to seek assistance, it's probably a good idea to do so.

If your loved one's primary care physician does not specialize in geriatric medicine, it may be time to seek out a doctor with this specialty. Geriatricians focus on the care and treatment of older persons, and they have a depth of understanding and experience with age-related diseases, including Alzheimer's. They will recognize the symptoms of normal aging and have the ability to differentiate them from organ decline and the development of diseases of the elderly. A geriatrician also will manage treatment of multiple medical disorders and the medications prescribed for each.

Treatments

The U.S. Food and Drug Administration has approved four medications for treatment of the symptoms of Alzheimer's disease. None of these medications will cure the disease, but they will slow the progression of symptoms for a period of time. (A fifth medication, Cognex, is no longer prescribed.)

In chapter 1, you read about the way neurons and synapses work in the brain to communicate with one another, and how Alzheimer's disease disrupts the neurotransmitters that send information from one brain cell to the next. Brain function becomes increasingly difficult as communication pathways become disabled and die.

Three of the four Alzheimer's medications—Aricept (donepezil), Razadyne (galantamine), and Exelon (rivastigmine)—are cholinesterase inhibitors. These drugs increase the brain's production of acetylcholine, a neurotransmitter required for neurons to communicate properly. With more acetylcholine moving between neurons, patients become more alert and their memories improve. Cholinesterase inhibitors achieve results in patients with mild to moderate Alzheimer's disease (though Aricept is FDA-approved for moderate to severe Alzheimer's), so their use will depend on the progression of the illness to date.

The fifth medication is Namenda (memantine), which works quite differently. This drug is an NMDA receptor antagonist, and it works by regulating a chemical called glutamate that occurs naturally in the brain. Damaged brain cells—whether affected by Alzheimer's disease or another brain disorder, such as vascular dementia—release large quantities of glutamate in the brain. Glutamate attaches to material called NMDA (N-methyl-D-aspartate) on the surface of brain cells, which allows calcium to flow into the cells. Too much calcium can accelerate the damage to these cells. Memantine protects the brain cells against this glutamate bombardment by blocking the NMDA receptors. Doctors prescribe Namenda for patients with moderate to severe Alzheimer's disease and related dementias, to help these patients retain their independence by maintaining daily functions for a few months longer than they would without the medication. You may appreciate the benefits of this prescription as much as your loved one, particularly when he can dress himself or use the bathroom independently.

Each of these drugs is usually prescribed for six months to one year, and only about half of the people who take them see any positive effect.

If the doctor chooses one of these drugs as a method of treatment, ask about the side effects of the specific medication. While most patients find the side effects to be fairly mild and short-lived, it's possible that your loved one will have a more severe reaction. You may need to decide if the improvement in cognitive function is worth the adverse effects (which can include nausea, diarrhea, indigestion, abdominal pain, and weight loss from loss of appetite).

The Alzheimer's Association almost always seeks volunteers for clinical trials to test new medications that may have a broader and more lasting effect or that may treat the underlying disease instead of the symptoms. To find out about these trials and determine your loved one's eligibility, visit the Alzheimer's Association Research Center website at www.alz.org/research/clinical_trials/clinical_trials_alzheimers.asp. You will be prompted to create an account and a profile before you can search for clinical trials currently in progress.

To date, no memory-enhancing herb or other natural substance has been tested extensively for its effectiveness in treating Alzheimer's disease and related dementias. Ginkgo biloba and huperzine A, widely promoted as effective treatments against Alzheimer's, have been disproved as a remedy for the disease in Phase 3 clinical trials. Omega-3 fatty acids have been proven to be slightly effective against normal age-related memory loss but not as a treatment for Alzheimer's.

Medication Management

In addition to Alzheimer's-specific drugs, your loved one may require medications for symptoms caused by the disease, but not controlled by the drugs described above. Symptoms can include depression, aggressive behavior, hallucinations or delusions, and disrupted or flipped sleep schedule (sleeping by day and wandering the house at night).

To treat these symptoms, your doctor may prescribe antidepressants or psychotropic drugs. The doctor may choose drugs used for epilepsy, not because seizures are expected, but because they can modify behavior. Sleeping medications can help get your loved one's circadian rhythms back on track, so you can both sleep through the night.

Finally, if your loved one is more than sixty-five years old, he or she probably has more physical conditions besides Alzheimer's that require medication. Perhaps he has high blood pressure, high cholesterol, a cardiac arrhythmia (irregular heartbeat), or respiratory or prostate issues. A female patient may take a preventive breast cancer drug or any number of other medications. Each of these has its own dosage, schedule, and requirements.

Inform the primary care doctor of every medication your loved one takes, both over-the-counter and prescription. The more pills your loved one has to swallow every day, the greater the chance of conflicts between one medication and another.

Managing all of these pills can be a daily challenge. To help you keep track of them, buy weeklong pill containers that have space for multiple daily doses: morning, noon, evening, and before bed. You'll also want to maintain an updated list of all medications and their dosages and the time of day at which each of them must be administered. Keep this schedule on your computer, and print out a complete list on the same day every week (on Sunday morning, for example); it will come in handy.

Load all of the medications into the pill containers. When you give your loved one the pills—and see that they have been swallowed—check them off your list, and note the time taken. You will have an easy reference for the next doctor appointment, and you can rest assured that all medications have been administered at the right time.

It's also important to inform your primary care doctor of every medication your loved one takes, both over-the-counter and prescription. The more pills taken, the better the chances that there will be conflicts between one medication and another. Duplication of effect also can happen when one doctor prescribes a drug to treat the same condition as another doctor. The result may not be dangerous, but there may be no additional benefit (and an unnecessary expense).

Making sure your loved one takes the medications can be a daily challenge. Alzheimer's patients often refuse medication for a variety of reasons that seem illogical or unapparent to caregivers: They may believe that you are trying to poison them, or that the medication will make them sick. Taking pills may become part of an elaborate delusion that frightens them. They may believe themselves to be perfectly healthy, so they can't understand why they need to take medication. Later in the course of the disease, they may simply not understand what the pills are or what they are to do with them. There are a number of solutions to this dilemma, including:

1. Never give a handful of pills to the patient. Hand them one pill at a time and let them swallow that one before giving another.

2. Try not to engage in arguments or long explanations of the need for the pills. Lots of discussion only confuses your loved one further.

3. Redirect their attention. Talk about something else while you hand them the pill and they swallow it.

4. If swallowing is a problem for your loved one, open the capsule and pour out the contents (or grind up the pill) and mix it into applesauce or pudding.

5. After they take the pills, give them positive reinforcement: a cup of their favorite soft drink or coffee, a snack, or something else they enjoy.

....

Some pills cannot be crushed or chewed, because disassembling the pill changes the way the medication works—particularly for time-release medications. Talk with your pharmacist or a registered nurse in your doctor's office (or your home health care agency, if you are using one) to determine if it's safe to crush up a specific pill. There may be a liquid form of the medication, and some pharmacies provide a choice of flavor additives to make them more palatable.

....

Physical Therapy

Both physical and occupational therapy can help improve your loved one's ability to function independently. In the early stages of Alzheimer's disease, therapists focus on improving balance and mobility, with an emphasis on preventing falls, getting up from a chair or bed, getting into and out of a car, and maintaining overall physical strength.

You may have the choice of bringing your loved one to a senior outpatient facility, such as a rehabilitation center, for physical and occupational therapy, or of having a therapist come to your home on a regular basis. If the therapist visits, he or she will help you change the environment to remove hazards and make it easier for your loved one to function in this space. The therapist will advise you on labeling drawers and cupboards, removing area rugs and other obstacles, clearing out visual clutter to help the Alzheimer's patient locate things she uses regularly, and make other modifications that may help your loved one stay in his own home for months or even years longer than you anticipated.

As the disease progresses, different kinds of physical and occupational therapy may help your family member. An occupational therapist can show you ways to make bathing, using the bathroom, dressing, and eating easier both for you and your loved one. While you know that she may be beyond the capacity to learn new things, you will be able to direct the action of your loved one to help make these personal hygiene activities go more smoothly.

The physical therapist has a role even as your loved one becomes less aware. Light exercise still helps with balance and mobility, so exercises in a chair or standing next to a wall can keep muscles functional and help your loved one continue to move around the space in relative safety.

Nearly all elderly people experience changes in their joints, whether they have some minor stiffness or develop arthritis; these changes can produce pain, which reduces mobility or the desire to move. In addition, bone density changes as people age, and issues like osteoporosis can lead to fractures and breakages. The best remedy is probably the one that feels the least likely: exercise can slow or even prevent these issues, and physical therapists are best equipped to convince an elderly person to move a stiffening joint on a regular basis.

The Health Insurance Portability and Accountability Act of 1996, or HIPAA, requires medical personnel to have permission in writing from their patients to discuss their medical issues with family members.

Tips for Successful Medical Visits

✓ **Get the HIPAA release signed.** The Health Insurance Portability and Accountability Act of 1996, or HIPAA, requires medical personnel to have permission in writing from their patients to discuss their medical issues with family members. You can get the form from your doctor's office. Officially, you need to have this signed before you can enter a doctor's exam room with your loved one, though most doctors will permit a caregiver who is also a family member to enter.

✓ **Inform the doctor before the visit.** When you make the appointment, tell the receptionist or nurse that your loved one has Alzheimer's disease. This will alert the doctor to the need for you to be in the exam room.

✓ **Be prepared.** Keep a list of questions for the doctor as they occur to you, and bring the list along to the appointment.

✓ **Allow enough time.** Leave for the appointment early enough to have time to transfer your loved one into the car, and to park and bring him into the doctor's office. You may need additional time to fill out paperwork as well if you're seeing a new doctor to whom you've been referred.

✓ **Know medications.** Bring your updated list of medications, including over-the-counter drugs, vitamins, and prescriptions from other doctors.

✓ **Go into the exam room with your loved one.** You need to hear what the doctor has to say in person, and you have questions of your own to ask. Even a healthy patient can have trouble remembering what the doctor tells him, so do not assume that your afflicted loved one will remember anything about the appointment, including instructions from the doctor.

✓ **Bring a pad and pen.** Take notes of the doctor's diagnoses and instructions. The doctor may give you a sheet of information before you leave, but you may hear him or her say things that are not on the sheet.

✓ **Make sure you understand what the doctor says.** Some physicians use a lot of technical medical language when they discuss a patient's case. Don't be afraid to stop the doctor and ask for clarification.

✓ **Let your loved one run the appointment.** Even though you are in the room, it's still your loved one's doctor, so she is officially in charge of the checkup or examination. You may meet with resistance or anger from your family member if you talk over her or if she has no opportunity to answer questions or tell the doctor how she feels. Don't jump in to answer questions right away; let her speak for himself as best she can. You can always fill in the missing details later.

✓ **Tell the doctor to address your loved one.** Again, it's easy to talk around the patient as if she were not in the room, but this only makes her feel helpless, as if her identity has already been lost. If the doctor immediately directs questions to you, say politely, "This is my mother's appointment, so please direct your questions to her. I'll help out when she needs me."

....

According to a study conducted in the emergency department of a hospital in Hong Kong, 29 percent of all accidents involving an elderly person at home took place in the bathroom, compared with only 14 percent in the kitchen. Seventy-five percent of all injuries were the result of falls, while the remaining 25 percent involved sharp objects, foreign body ingestion, crush injuries, and burning or scalding (just 3 percent).

....

CHAPTER FIVE

Safety First

Whether you are looking out for your loved one with Alzheimer's disease in his own home or you've moved him into your house, you need to make some changes to the environment to make it as safe as possible.

Alzheimer's affects a number of cognitive functions that we all take for granted, and these in turn can affect good judgment, behavior, and the ability to move through a familiar space. Perhaps your loved one does not remember to turn off the stove or how to handle an iron or a screwdriver safely. Patients may not recognize their own belongings or remember which room is the bedroom, even if they have slept in that room for decades. Familiar objects suddenly appear unfamiliar, and people who have been friends or family members throughout their lifetime may arouse fear or suspicion.

On top of the hazards that come along with dementia, your loved one most likely experiences the basic changes that come with aging. She may have balance issues that require the use of a cane or walker. Her hearing or vision may have declined significantly, requiring hearing aides and bifocal glasses—both of which an Alzheimer's patient may repeatedly misplace. Accompanying these changes may be difficulty with depth perception or greater than normal trouble seeing at night.

All of these issues can turn an environment you once considered safe into a dangerous obstacle course. Alzheimer's patients have continuous cognitive impairment, so it can be tough to predict what your loved one might do next. A room that seemed safe this morning can contain a number of hazards by evening, simply because your loved one no longer remembers that the stove is hot, or because he feels an inexplicable need to take the toaster apart. Your best bet is to adapt your environment as much as possible to remove the potential for accidents, and watch closely to see what new issues may arise on a daily basis. Here are some ways to make your living space safer for your loved one.

....

Alzheimer's patients have continuous cognitive impairment, so it can be tough to predict what they might do next. A room that seemed safe this morning can contain a number of hazards by evening.

....

Home Safety

Walk through the rooms of your home and take a good look at the traffic patterns and the placement of furniture and other objects. What might get in the way of a person who has trouble perceiving his surroundings? Remove every tripping hazard: throw rugs, piles of newspapers and magazines, coffee tables and end tables that partially obstruct doorways or jut into the walkway, and frayed ends of carpeting that need tacking down. Most people become so used to walking around things that they barely realize these obstacles are there, so you may want to make this walk-through with a friend or home health professional who can spot things you overlook.

Check the doors that lead outside or that go into parts of your home that are not conducive to an Alzheimer's patient. Keep doors that go outside locked to reduce the possibility of your loved one wandering away. You might consider installing an alarm system, if you don't already have one. Your garage, basement, attic, and even your kitchen may not be safe places for your loved one, especially as the disease advances and cognitive symptoms become more pronounced.

The Alzheimer's Association suggests disguising doors that lead outside or to places that may be dangerous so your loved one does not recognize them. Cover doors with a cloth, a screen, or a painted mural, or use swinging or folding doors to replace doors with knobs—essentially disguising these objects. This may be enough to discourage an Alzheimer's patient from trying to go through.

At the end of this chapter, you'll find a checklist of areas and items to secure in order to make your home as safe as possible for your loved one. It's a delicate balance between maintaining a livable, relaxed home for you and your family and keeping your Alzheimer's patient safe, but minimizing the potential for accidents does help create a more comfortable home for everyone who lives there.

Personal Safety

With so much of your time spent focused on your loved one's safety, you may do one of the most common things that caregivers do: neglect your own safety.

Protecting yourself from injury is every bit as important as taking care of your family member with Alzheimer's disease. Back and shoulder injuries are very common among caregivers, because they are often challenged to lift as much as their own body weight while transferring the person from a bed to a chair or from a wheelchair to the toilet. Lifting and turning improperly can result in debilitating conditions that will not only cause you great pain but also make it impossible for you to continue in your caregiver role.

While you may feel that you are managing fairly well, the physical impact becomes cumulative due to the daily repetition of these tasks. You may be injuring disks and muscles in your back over time, so that by the time you feel the sudden, severe pain of a ruptured disk, the damage could be extensive.

Talk with your doctor or your home health care agency, if you are using one, about the safest methods for lifting and turning a patient. If you are taking your loved one to physical therapy, ask the therapist to teach you how to do these things safely.

The devices that you install in your bedroom, bathroom, and other rooms to help your loved one transfer himself can also take much of the strain off of your body. Grab bars, handles on toilet seats, benches in showers, and recliners that lift your loved one to a standing position allow him to assist in the transfer or even complete some of the transfers on his own with your supervision.

If it takes two people to lift your loved one, Medicare may pay for the rental of a portable Hoyer lift, a sling lift or sit-to-stand lift that uses hydraulic power to help people with mobility, which will make it possible for you alone to assist your loved one in getting up off the floor or out of bed. Talk to your doctor about writing a prescription for the lift.

Patient Safety Precautions

Beyond taking precautions to prevent falls and accidents, you can guard against a number of other issues that can put Alzheimer's patients—and many other seniors—in danger at home.

- **Food and drink temperature.** The ability to sense heat and cold diminishes as people get older. When serving coffee, tea, soup, or hot food to your loved one, keep the temperature no higher than about 120 degrees Fahrenheit to prevent burns.

- **Staying home alone.** Is it safe to leave a person with Alzheimer's alone at home? There's no simple answer to this question, as it has to do with the advancement of the disease and the person's cognitive abilities. If your loved one becomes agitated or withdrawn when left alone, or if he is likely to become disoriented when alone and attempt to wander, it would be unwise to leave him unsupervised.

- **Emergencies.** Many people with moderate to severe Alzheimer's forget what to do in an emergency, so if they find themselves in a dangerous situation, they do not know how to call the police or the fire department (even if the instructions are hanging by the phone).

- **Driving.** People in the early stages of Alzheimer's may be able to drive, but over time they will lose the quick reflexes and decision-making capabilities that driving requires. When your loved one reaches this stage, it's time to take away the car keys and sell the car, no matter how much the person objects. This is a tough conversation to have with your loved one, as the lack of ability to drive signals the end of independence—but for the person's own safety and the safety of others on the road, it has to be done. Be gentle but firm when you discuss this decision with your loved one. If all else fails, ask the person's doctor for a letter that states that it has become dangerous for her to drive. If your loved one respects the doctor's authority, it may bring the discussion to a quick conclusion.

- **Watch for unsupervised activity.** Alzheimer's patients may try to do things they did before they became ill, some of which—cooking or using tools, for example—become hazardous in short order when the person loses track in the middle of the process.

- **Discourage solicitors.** People with Alzheimer's are particularly vulnerable to credit-card companies, contests, nonprofit fund-raising calls, and other solicitations. You can avoid contact with some of these by setting all phone calls at home to go to voicemail on the first ring, keeping your loved one from answering the phone. Hang a "No Solicitations" sign at your door.

- **Seek professional help.** As much as you want to help your loved one in every possible way, there may be tasks for which you simply do not have enough information or training. For example, your family member's advancing Alzheimer's disease may lead to a need for tube feeding, a procedure for which nursing training would be appropriate. If you agree to take on such a responsibility without a full understanding of the skills and techniques involved, the result could be harmful to your loved one. If you know that you are out of your depth, it's time to look into alternatives: home health care by a professional aide or nurse, or relocation of your loved one to a skilled nursing facility (see chapter 12 for more information). This is not a failure on your part. It's simply the reality of the disease, and you must do what will be best, both for the patient and for you.

If you know that you are out of your depth, it's time to look into alternatives: home health care by a professional aide or nurse, or relocation of your loved one to a skilled nursing facility. This is not a failure on your part.

Safety Checklist

✓ Have a list of emergency phone numbers ready on your smartphone or near your home phone.

✓ Check fire extinguishers, smoke detectors, carbon monoxide detectors, and any other devices to be sure they're in working order. Change the batteries every six months.

✓ Install deadbolt locks on doors.

✓ Add lights in hallways and entryways, and leave a nightlight on in the bathrooms.

✓ If your stairways are not carpeted, place adhesive, non-skid strips on the stair treads.

✓ Store guns in locked boxes, and place the keys where the Alzheimer's patient cannot find them. Install safety locks on the guns, and remove ammunition and firing pins when storing the guns. The Alzheimer's Association recommends removing guns from the house altogether to prevent an unexpected accident.

✓ Lock up power tools and other machinery in your garage, basement, or in cabinets in your workspace.

✓ Lock up medications, and take them out only to dispense them.

✓ Clear floors of piles of magazines, newspapers, laundry, shoes, or anything else that may cause someone to trip.

✓ Check carpets for loose edges that can catch a foot or a walker, and tack these down firmly.

- ✓ Put decals on sliding glass doors at eye level.

- ✓ Put away remote controls when they are not in use.

- ✓ Put childproof locks on cabinet doors that contain anything breakable, poisonous, or dangerous.

- ✓ Store hazardous chemicals out of your loved one's reach, preferably in a locked cabinet.

- ✓ Place a lock on your liquor cabinet or wine rack, or put the liquor or wine in a cabinet out of reach.

- ✓ Disguise or lock doors to restrict access to basements, attics, and other areas that may contain hazardous materials, tools, chemicals, and dark staircases.

- ✓ Remove locks from bathroom doors to keep the person with Alzheimer's from locking himself inside. If you need a lock for your own privacy, get one that you can unlock from the outside.

- ✓ Install grab bars in the tub and shower, and a seat with handrails on the toilet.

- ✓ Use a single faucet that mixes hot and cold water in the tub and sink, to reduce the possibility of hot water burns.

- ✓ Place slip-proofing strips or decals on the bottom of the shower and tub and in front of the bathroom sink.

- ✓ Set your water heater's temperature to 120 degrees Fahrenheit to avoid burns.

- ✓ Have an automatic shut-off switch and safety knobs installed on your stove.

- ✓ Remove objects (magnets, novelty candles, plastic fruit) that can be mistaken for food.

- ✓ If smoking is permitted in your home, keep matches and lighters out of sight when not in use.

- ✓ Keep your cars locked and in the garage.

✓ If you haven't done so upon diagnosis, stop allowing your loved one to drive.

✓ If the person with Alzheimer's used tools for work, he may attempt to do so again. Keep your tools in locked cabinets, and put away any items (small appliances, for example) that you do not want taken apart.

CHAPTER SIX

Behavioral Changes and Care

Memory loss is just one symptom of Alzheimer's disease. As the condition progresses, a person with dementia will begin to exhibit behavioral changes that may be disconcerting and troubling to watch. Some of these behaviors also may be socially inappropriate.

As a caregiver, your first impulse may be to try to stop the behavior that you find troubling. If continuing the behavior will place the person or others in danger, or if it could lead to something that could be considered indecent, then bringing a quick end to the behavior may be the right thing to do. If it's merely peculiar, however, there may be no harm in letting it continue.

This chapter will help you understand the behaviors you see and what each behavior says about the progress of the disease. It also provides some advice about ways to limit or stop actions that could injure or expose your loved one in ways that are incompatible with their situation.

The Seven Stages of Alzheimer's Disease

The stages, symptoms, and progression of Alzheimer's can vary greatly from patient to patient. Barry Reisberg, MD, clinical director of the New York University School of Medicine's Silberstein Aging and Dementia Research Center, developed seven stages to identify how a person's abilities change throughout the course of the disease. Based on his framework, the Alzheimer's Association defines these seven stages of the disease:

STAGE 1: NO IMPAIRMENT

The person shows no symptoms of dementia. A medical professional will not be able to detect any evidence of symptoms of dementia.

STAGE 2: VERY MILD COGNITIVE DECLINE

The person may forget familiar words or misplace things like keys and glasses. Friends and family notice nothing amiss, and doctors do not see signs of dementia.

STAGE 3: MILD DECLINE

Difficulty retrieving a name or word, trouble remembering new information, and struggling to do simple things all can be early signs of Alzheimer's disease. The person may lose things that are valuable or have trouble keeping a schedule or planning activities.

STAGE 4: MODERATE DECLINE

Symptoms become more obvious at this point: forgetting recent visits from family or events the person attended, difficulty with complex tasks (like managing finances), forgetting things in their own history, or withdrawing from social situations because of confusion or an inability to follow conversation.

STAGE 5: MODERATELY SEVERE DECLINE

The person needs help with everyday activities like choosing clothing to wear or with taking care of things around the house. They have trouble with arithmetic or can't recall their own telephone number or address. Days and times become confusing and hard to remember; they may not know what day or month it is when asked. At this point, the person can still eat and use the bathroom without assistance.

STAGE 6: SEVERE DECLINE

This is the stage at which major personality and behavior changes take place. Patients may remember their own name, but not the names of others, and their personal history may become a blur. They can tell a familiar face from someone they have never met, but do not know the name of the familiar person. A person at this stage needs help with activities of daily living, including dressing, bathing, and using the bathroom, and they may sleep through the day and wander at night. Wandering in general becomes a risk. Delusions and paranoia—believing that people are not who they say they are or that they are in danger—and hallucinations—seeing people and things that are not there—are possible. Repetitive behaviors are common.

STAGE 7: VERY SEVERE DECLINE

At this stage, patients can no longer respond to the environment. They need assistance with every aspect of daily care and hygiene, and they may have involuntary movement, incontinence, and an inability to sit without support.

Your loved one may seem to fit into several stages. Most people have a myriad of symptoms from several different stages, making it hard to determine where they are in the Alzheimer's spectrum.

Behavior Changes in the Early Stages (Stages 1 to 4)

It's easy to become focused on lapses in memory as the first clue that your loved one may have Alzheimer's disease, but many other behavioral changes can signal the onset of this condition as well.

Simple things that used to be routine for your family member may suddenly become very difficult: Your mother used a computer every day at work and now can't seem to get into her email account. Your father worked with tools throughout his career and now can't make his screwdriver work. When pressed, your parent offers a long list of logical explanations for the lapse in skill. After checking these routine reasons—a problem with the Internet, or other medical issues contributing to muscle weakness or vision—these changes are likely signs that dementia has begun.

Simple daily tasks—cooking a meal, using a can opener, turning on the clothes washer, using the telephone, dusting and vacuuming the house, using the TV remote control, washing the dishes, handling money—can become complicated and mysterious to a person with Alzheimer's disease. The change may begin with a single task and spread to others over time.

Your loved one is unlikely to tell you these things are happening, but you will become aware of them as they develop. Perhaps you will begin receiving phone calls from your family member telling you that their computer isn't working or that the remote control is broken. If you visit and try to "fix" whatever is broken, you may find nothing wrong at all.

Getting impatient, questioning, or confronting your loved one at this point is counterproductive; the dread of finding out that they are developing a dementia is exactly why they do not want to tell you when something is wrong. Their reaction may well be defensive, repeating the long list of reasons why the remote or the computer didn't work.

One of the most frustrating parts of dealing with a relative in the early stages of Alzheimer's disease is also one of the most poignant. Your loved one does not want to tell you that she has trouble with things that used to be second nature, because they know what comes next: loss of independence. Despite the cognitive problems that have come to light, your loved one will deny, rationalize, and make excuses for her inability to perform basic tasks—and all of these excuses will seem plausible. As long as only one, two, or a few things seem to be amiss, she can continue to make you question your own judgment about the changes you are certain are taking place.

Eventually, however, these changes will pile up. You will see a pattern of behavior that will warrant further evaluation:

- Lack of interest in food

- Loss of energy

- Disinterest in cleaning the house, doing laundry, or doing dishes

- Struggle to learn new information

- Leaving spoiled food in the refrigerator

- Desire to stay home rather than see friends or family

- Insomnia

At this point, your loved one can continue to live independently with some assistance—and that assistance may be as basic as a daily phone call from you. Your role is not so much full-time caregiver as facilitator, helping your loved one remain at home and be part of the decision-making process for what lies ahead.

Managing Early-Stage Behavioral Changes

- **Maintain independence.** Encourage your loved one to continue to live in her home for as long as she can. In these familiar surroundings, your loved one can remain safe and comfortable and retain self-confidence.

- **Visit as often as you can—every day if possible.** If you can't visit regularly, put together a team of people who can: your siblings, your loved one's siblings, a close friend, or other family members. Take note of what has changed and what may not be getting done around the house.

- **Provide assistance with cleaning.** Your loved one may resist having a cleaning service or even letting you tidy up. Try involving her in the process of choosing a service. If necessary, enlist a friend or sibling to take the person with Alzheimer's out for an afternoon while you clean the house or have it cleaned.

- **Provide assistance with meals.** Many metropolitan areas have services like Meals on Wheels that bring nutritious meals to seniors at home. If this is not an option, try to choose simple recipes with your loved one so she can continue to do her own cooking. Take her grocery shopping regularly to be sure there is fresh food in the house, and clean out the refrigerator every week to get rid of spoiled foods.

- **Pay the bills.** Many people with Alzheimer's or related dementia give up writing checks and paying bills very early in the disease's progression. With online bill paying and direct withdrawals, you can automate a great deal of this process. If you prefer to write out checks, collect your family member's mail on a weekly basis and write checks from her account for her to sign. Perhaps your loved one will feel most comfortable sitting with you as you do this, so she knows exactly where the money is going.

- **Eliminate unnecessary tasks.** If your loved one can't keep the garden tools straight or struggles to pick out flowers to plant in spring, planting may be a task you can eliminate altogether. Look for other tasks that just don't need doing, like sewing and ironing.

Behavior Changes in the Moderate to Severe Stages (Stages 5 to 7)

Not all people with Alzheimer's disease have the same symptoms, but many do experience behavioral changes that can be both challenging and upsetting to you in your role as a caregiver.

Your loved one may have trouble sleeping, wandering the house at night when the rest of the family is in bed. She may have verbal outbursts, or become agitated and lash out to hit or kick you. She may become restless, pacing in one room or moving around the house in a repetitive pattern.

Some Alzheimer's patients shred paper, pull apart cotton or pillow stuffing, hang paper towels around the house, or repeatedly take everything out of a wallet and put it back in. They may pack and unpack a suitcase over and over, or take everything out of a drawer and put it back in, only to take it all out again. These behaviors all stem from anxiety, a sense that they have to do something important or find a missing item, but they can't remember what.

If the repetitive behavior is not hurting your loved one or you, there may be no reason to attempt to stop it. If you see signs that they are agitated or anxious, however, talk to them calmly and gently, and find out what they may be looking for or thinking they have to do. You may be able to alleviate the anxiety and redirect it into a less disturbing behavior.

Some patients with severe Alzheimer's disease become agitated for no immediately apparent reason—but there is almost always some trigger. The person may simply be bored or tired, or they may not feel well. Too much caffeine can cause irritability and anger as well as restlessness; so limiting the number of cups of coffee can help to decrease these issues. Check to see if your loved one needs to use the bathroom, another situation that can cause agitation if they cannot find the words to express the need.

....

Something as simple as closing the door to the room and blocking out the noise and commotion can reduce anxiety and agitation.

....

Managing Moderate- to Severe-Stage Behavioral Changes

- **Be patient and calm.** As long as the person is not in danger, there's no need to react with great urgency.

- **Communicate in a normal, calm voice.** Shouting at or berating your loved one will not "snap" her into reality.

- **Use loving words.** Never tell your loved one that she is stupid or crazy.

- **Don't attempt to tell the person that he's wrong.** All this does is create more anxiety and agitation.

- **Listen to what the person is saying.** Sometimes you can pick up clues that tell you why this behavior is taking place. These clues will help you find a solution.

- **Watch the behavior.** If this behavior is repeated on many occasions, try to determine what triggers it. Is it a television program, or something that happens every day at dinnertime, or when folding clothes or taking out the trash? Whatever it may be, a change in your own routine, behavior, or environment may prevent the trigger from continuing.

- **Reduce triggers in the environment.** Loud noise, sun glare, bright light, and too many people going in and out can all function as triggers. Something as simple as closing the door to the room and blocking out the noise and commotion can reduce anxiety and agitation.

- **Reduce clutter in the house.** The visual confusion of clutter can make the person with Alzheimer's more agitated.

- **Create a routine.** Have your meals at the same time every day, and make a specific bedtime. The repetition and predictability can be calming for your loved one.

CHAPTER SEVEN

Mental Changes and Care

Memory loss and confusion, two of the most prevalent and recognized symptoms of Alzheimer's disease, may develop so gradually that you and the person with the disease may not recognize them for what they are. Easy to excuse as the hazards of aging, the occasional misplacement of keys can be seen as trivial, and the stumble over a grandchild's name can be explained away and laughed off. As the memory loss progresses, however, there can be no further excuses as the person with Alzheimer's begins to lose the personal freedom and independence that they expected to enjoy through their last days on earth.

Very often, the person who has the disease knows exactly what has happened to her and what will continue to happen in the months and years to come. As a caregiver, you will be faced not only with your loved one's memory loss, confusion, and the onset of delusions and other distortions of reality but also with your own grappling with their depression, anxiety, fear, and sense of loss. The more you can anticipate and be prepared for these potential states of mind, the more effective you will be in your caregiver role.

What to Expect: Early Stages (1 to 4) Versus Late Stages (5 to 7)

Memory Loss

At first, changes in memory may seem like nothing more than normal age-related memory loss, perhaps with some unusual twists. Your loved one may forget information she recently learned, such as how to use a new phone or remote control, or the way to use a new appliance. She may forget a child's birthday or another important date, and you may discover lists tacked up all over the house, often with the same information on all of them. You may begin getting calls from Mom to help her with her computer or television, during which she insists that the device is "broken."

Over time, your loved one will begin to struggle with following instructions, like the steps in a recipe or the way to use a smartphone. She may falter in handling her own finances because she can no longer add columns of numbers or balance a checkbook. Your loved one may become confused over time and place, not realizing that you live hundreds of miles away or that it's summer or winter. By the time you get a call from a friend (or the police) saying that your loved one has lost her way in her own neighborhood, you can no longer hope that what you've seen is just normal age-related memory loss.

When your loved one's condition moves from mild to moderate, you will see significant changes in cognitive abilities. She may not be able to judge distance or understand visual information and may struggle to find the right word to express a thought, substituting another word—often one that seems nonsensical—for the one she wanted. Your loved one may call people and things by the wrong name, including members of the family, or forget names of loved ones altogether. Misplacing things results from putting normal things in abnormal places, like putting gloves in the freezer or hiding pencils under a rug. People in later stages may ransack a room looking for something they believe is missing, and then have no memory of making the mess. When they can't find these things later, they may decide that a robbery has taken place.

Some of these memory issues will lead to changes in personality. A normally fastidious gentleman may wear the same clothes for days and refuse to change or to bathe. Small upsets may generate incompatibly large reactions—what the medical community calls "catastrophic reactions"—to such things as an object being moved to a new place or a wallet ending up in the wrong compartment of a shoulder bag. Confusion, anxiety, and fear become common reactions to situations that have never been problems before. Eventually, delusions may make the person with Alzheimer's believe that people around them are plotting against them, hiding their belongings, or deliberately snubbing them. They may feel urgency that no one else feels—a certainty that something is terribly wrong.

Hallucinations

The act of hallucinating involves actually seeing or hearing things that are not real. People with hallucinations may see a deceased relative in the room—most commonly a spouse—or they may hear people whispering racial slurs or insults as they pass them in a hallway or a store. They may see the people in a television show actually sitting in the room with them. In some cases, hallucinations become elaborate: they may see a wedding taking place in the next room, for example, or they may see a real person transform into something terrifying. You may see your loved one talking to people who are not there, or trying to collect objects or animals that you do not see.

Delusions

Different than hallucinations, delusions involve feelings, suspicions, or confused information that your loved one makes sense of by creating a new version of reality. They may be suspicious of other people, believe that they are being held prisoner, or determine that your home is their place of business. Delusions may cause people to feel a sense of urgency when nothing is actually wrong. You may find them searching the house for "the baby," or practicing a compulsive behavior that they believe will keep him safe.

The possibilities for these hallucinations and delusions are as unlimited as the cognitive dysfunctions of the people who have them. While not all Alzheimer's patients have hallucinations and delusions, many do develop these distortions of reality in the late stages of the disease.

If the changes come on suddenly, they may not be caused by a dramatic change in your family member's disease. Pneumonia and urinary tract infections are both common causes of a pronounced cognitive change in elderly people, especially when the change triggers hallucinations. Start by having your loved one evaluated by your primary care physician to rule out an infection as the cause.

If there's no infection and the behavior and psychiatric changes are indeed the result of Alzheimer's disease, look for changes in your loved one's environment that may have triggered this extreme response. Has the person recently made a major move to a new place, or has there been a change in his caregiver? Spending time in the hospital, having guests in the house, or something as basic as a change in routine all can trigger major behavioral shifts.

What should you do when your loved one has these hallucinations or delusions?

- **Don't try to convince your loved one that they are wrong** or that reality is not what it seems. In many cases, this only makes the person angry or more agitated as she tries to convince you otherwise.

- **Go along with the perception and take it to a conclusion.** Let's say your mother believes that she works at your house and wants to know when she will be paid. You might like to retort that you're the one doing all the work and she has a lot of nerve, but this will only end in an argument, which will not accomplish anything useful. Instead, try telling her, "Your paychecks are being direct-deposited right into your bank account." You have taken her perception to its logical end, and she will most likely be satisfied—and there's no argument and no hurt feelings. Chances are that you can apply this method to many situations with your loved one.

- **Redirect the person's focus onto something less threatening.** Suggest an activity that your loved one enjoys, or make an offer of food or drink. Coax her into a different room to move her away from a television or radio that may be causing the issue. Suggest some exercise: Go for a walk together, or have her help you with a simple chore, like folding laundry. The specific redirection that works for your loved one may be entirely different, but the important thing is to refocus her attention away from whatever has triggered the episode, and onto something more benign.

If hallucinations, delusions, and disruptive behavior persist, or if you fear that your loved one may harm someone, it's time to consider medication as a partial solution. Antidepressants can help to relieve irritability and depression, and antianxiety medication (anxiolytics) can reduce restlessness and disruptive behavior. Antipsychotic drugs, used carefully and under a doctor's supervision, can alleviate these symptoms and return some normalcy to your loved one's days. A group of these antipsychotic medications called "atypical" drugs, however, have been shown to increase the risk of stroke and death in older people with dementia, according to the U.S. Food and Drug Administration. It's up to you to decide if this risk is appropriate in calming your loved one's symptoms.

Confusion

With memory loss comes confusion, a condition that increases as Alzheimer's disease progresses. Confusion is a broad term that covers all kinds of symptoms of the disease:

- Impaired perception of time and place

- Inability to identify people the patient knows well

- Uncertainty about a common object: what it is and what it is for

- Getting lost while walking or driving

- Inability to recognize the patient's own home

- Belief that a grown child is a baby

- Ideas that deceased people are living

- Inability to remember the patient's own name

- Lack of understanding about an activity going on around them

....

If you can respond to the fear by taking calm, comforting action, you may be able to break a cycle of confusion for long enough to alleviate some of your loved one's stress.

....

As your loved one moves from moderate to severe Alzheimer's, these symptoms become more pronounced. The lack of recognition of familiar people can lead to emotional outbursts such as yells for help, or insistence that you are lying about who you are and what you're doing there.

These times can be painful to observe, especially if you are someone who has been close with your loved one throughout your life. Imagine, however, how terrifying this confusion can be to this patient, who does not know who all these strangers are or why these people insist on doing things for her and to her. If you can respond to the fear by taking calm, comforting action, you may be able to break a cycle of confusion for long enough to alleviate some of your loved one's stress.

At the end of this chapter, you'll find a list of ways to respond to your loved one's confusion and accompanying fear.

Emotional Care

Just as your loved one has physical needs met through nutritious meals, comfortable surroundings, proper hygiene, and ample sleep, so should she have her emotional needs met. Alzheimer's patients may not have the same cognitive abilities they enjoyed throughout their lifetime, but they still require companionship, affection, and meaningful activities that provide a sense of usefulness and accomplishment.

The Eden Alternative, a revolutionary elder care philosophy that has transformed many senior living communities across the country, begins with a basic tenet: "The three plagues of loneliness, helplessness, and boredom account for the bulk of suffering among our elders." In addition to the burdens of Alzheimer's disease and its ability to steal memories and identity, your loved one faces the last years of life with less ability to interact with friends and family, function independently and have control of daily life, and enjoy the activities that filled her days until this disease developed past the early stages.

Aging does not mean that your loved one suddenly likes listening to Lawrence Welk and playing bingo. At various times in life, your family member has pursued hobbies, managed a career, fixed things around the house, cooked, cleaned, raised children, enjoyed music and games, traveled to exotic places, and did any number of other things that made life rich and full. While Alzheimer's disease makes it more difficult to enjoy these activities in the conventional sense, your loved one's identity did not disappear with the damaged brain cells. She still will enjoy the things she has always enjoyed, with some modifications.

Gardening, taking pictures, feeding birds, watching sports, cleaning the house, baking cookies, corresponding with friends online—all of these activities can still be within reach for the person with Alzheimer's. The parameters of the activity may change to accommodate the extent of the person's memory loss, but the favorite pastime does not have to cease because of the person's new disability.

Give your loved one the opportunity to choose to do this favorite activity, within safe guidelines—but not so safe that she feels belittled or that you're treating her like a child. If possible, talk with her about ways you may need to modify the hobby, and come to a conclusion together.

Based on your discussion, your loved one may choose not to take up the favorite hobby for a number of reasons. Perhaps she understands that her ability to do this thing has been compromised, or maybe the advancement of the disease made her lose interest in things that used to fascinate her. If this pastime is no longer within reach, work with your loved one to find something else she might enjoy.

Friends and family members can become scarce when they do not understand the advancement of Alzheimer's disease and its impact on an individual's ability to communicate. People outside the caregiving circle may feel discomfort at coming to visit your loved one, even though they have been close for generations. They may fear that they will say or do something foolish, or that your loved one's behavior will be erratic. It's not uncommon for these people to disappear from your loved one's life just as she needs companionship and conversation most. Some will actually say to you, "I want to remember her the way she was, not the way she is now."

Encourage friends and family to come and visit anyway. Schedule the visit for a time when your family member is usually more clearheaded and less confused—for most Alzheimer's patients, this would be in the morning. Limit the guest list to just one or two people, and turn off the TV, music, or radio during the visit, so there will be just one voice at a time.

Tips for Visitors

If your visitors have no experience with dementia patients, it may be helpful to provide a few guidelines to help the visit go smoothly. (These may be good reminders for you as well.)

- ✓ **Speak slowly and clearly.** Language is often hard to use and grasp for people with Alzheimer's.

- ✓ **Sit where you will be face-to-face.** Facial expressions convey a lot of information that will help the person respond.

- ✓ **Begin by saying your loved one's name.** This will to get her attention before asking a question.

- ✓ **Expect a delay.** It will take your loved one longer than normal to process information and form a reply. There's no need to continue speaking to fill the gap until they reply; doing so may only frustrate your loved one.

- ✓ **Use short sentences and simple words.** This will ease anxiety as the patient searches for her words.

✓ **Watch your body language.** If you look exasperated or bored, or if you cross your arms over your chest, you may appear to be angry to the person with Alzheimer's.

✓ **Stay with familiar topics.** People with Alzheimer's have trouble taking in new information or learning new concepts, so this is not the time to discuss the latest new political issue or show her a new video game.

✓ **Be prepared for repetition.** The person with Alzheimer's will ask the same question or make the same statement more than once, and possibly repeatedly. For example, she may tell you, "Oh, you've changed your hairstyle," over and over again. Just keep giving the same answer with a smile; there's no need to point out to them that they are repeating the statement. This is out of their control.

✓ **Do not point out when she used the wrong word or has said something that doesn't make sense to you.** This is also beyond your loved one's control and correcting her will not make the word choice improve. It also may upset her. Instead, do your best to understand, and continue the conversation. You might also say, "I'm not quite following, but let's come back to that," or "I'm not very good at understanding this morning."

✓ **Keep your visit short.** Be aware of when the person appears to be tiring out, or when it seems that the conversation is more frustrating to her than beneficial.

Responding to Mental Confusion: Do's and Don'ts

■ **Do keep objects the person recognizes in her room.** Make sure these things are in view.

■ **Do place familiar photos of family and friends where your loved one can see them.** These can help calm her fears and improve orientation.

- **Do remove things from the room that the person does not need.** Too much clutter, especially with unfamiliar objects, can make a place seem foreign and confusing.

- **Do speak slowly and clearly.** Use nonthreatening words.

- **Do make sure the person looks at you while you talk.** Your calm, gentle facial expression is just as important as the words you say.

- **Do introduce yourself.** If the person does not recognize you, you need to reestablish trust every time you enter the room.

- **Do explain what you're going to do before you do it.** This makes your actions less frightening.

- **Do mute or turn off the television or radio when you come into the room.** This reduces noise confusion.

- **Do involve the person in decision making.** The more the person feels "done to," the more confused and threatened they will feel.

- **Do ask for feedback.** Ask your loved one how she feels, if the room is too warm, if she'd like to be in a different chair, and so on. This enhances the person's sense of control over her surroundings.

- **Do establish routines.** If the same thing happens at the same time every day, it becomes a touchstone that helps with orientation of time and place.

- **Don't berate or shout at the person.** Don't ask, "How can you not remember me?" People with Alzheimer's are not withholding affection; they have a degenerative brain disease that causes significant memory loss.

- **Don't use baby talk.** Your loved one is an adult, no matter how childlike her behavior may seem.

- **Don't correct her or dismiss her confusion.** Remember that these issues are very real and important to your loved one.

CHAPTER EIGHT

Challenges of the Daily Routine

Alzheimer's disease is a progressive illness, one that will result in the person with the disease needing assistance with all activities of daily living: bathing, dressing, eating, using the bathroom, and so on. In addition to the basic necessities, most Alzheimer's patients have trouble sleeping normally, often becoming unable to discern day from night. The transitional part of the day, from daylight to twilight, can trigger a phenomenon that medical professionals call "sundowning," a period of increased confusion, delusions, and even hallucinations for some Alzheimer's patients.

As you take on the caregiving role, one of the most beneficial things you can do is establish a daily routine, with specific times for various activities of daily living and structured pastimes in between. Adjust this routine as the person's needs change, taking into account her ability to assist in personal care activities and any changes in her preferences as she moves into the later stages of the disease. The more routine the day becomes, the better your chances of heading off repeated periods of sundowning and other confused or delusional behavior.

Eating

In all stages of Alzheimer's disease, maintaining proper nutrition helps keep a person's body healthy, which can help reduce behavioral issues in the shorter term. It also reduces the severity of a number of additional illnesses that can affect quality of life, such as heart disease and diabetes.

The basic elements of good nutrition do not vary a great deal throughout our lives, though recent changes in the federal guidelines for a balanced diet emphasize more foods from plant-based sources—fruits, vegetables, and whole grains—and fewer from animal-based sources, including meats, eggs, and dairy products. For people with Alzheimer's disease and anyone in the second half of life, a diet that contains low-fat dairy products and little saturated fat is more healthful for the heart. Avoid foods with high levels of fat and cholesterol, including fatty meat, butter and other solid fats, and whole milk.

Sodium has long been known to affect blood pressure, so substitute herbs and spices for salt in cooking. Do your best to avoid frozen dinners, canned soups, and other convenience foods that contain high levels of sodium.

The Alzheimer's Association recommends a reduction in refined sugars in a patient's diet; because these processed foods (cakes, cookies, candy) generally do not contain much, if any, nutritional value. However, if your loved one is in later-stage Alzheimer's and has little appetite, adding foods with refined sugar will do no further harm, and they may encourage her to eat more.

Why do Alzheimer's patients lose their appetites? Some issues may be directly related to their disease. People in the later stages of Alzheimer's may struggle to differentiate the food on their plate from the plate itself, or they may no longer recognize foods that have been favorites. The senses of smell and taste diminish as all people age, so foods may not taste the way they did before—or they may have no taste at all. Medications may reduce a patient's appetite as well, so if your loved one has started a new drug and you see a sudden drop in appetite, notify your doctor to see if there's an alternative.

Significant reductions in activity level also can cause a loss of appetite. Try to include some exercise in your loved one's day, whether it's a walk around the neighborhood, chair calisthenics, or housecleaning. Even a little bit of exercise can help burn calories and promote hunger. While older adults in general need fewer calories because of the decrease in their metabolism and a reduced amount of exercise, their nutritional needs remain much the same throughout their lives—so a balanced diet continues to be a high priority.

If your loved one has no appetite and begins to lose weight, your doctor may suggest adding nutritional supplement drinks (like Ensure or Boost) to the person's diet. You may prefer that your family get its nutrients from fresh food, but these supplements provide calories, vitamins, and minerals for people who have difficulty chewing or swallowing, or who have simply lost interest in eating.

....

Flavor comes from a combination of smelling and tasting. Our mouths have about nine thousand taste buds, which sense food that is sweet, salty, sour, or bitter. Other flavors come from the aroma of the food. All people lose taste buds as they get older, with salty and sweet tastes diminishing first, and sour and bitter disappearing later. If your loved one was a heavy smoker, or if she had a job in which she worked with harmful chemicals, she might lose the senses of smell and taste faster than average for an older person.

....

Tips For Helping Your Loved One Get Nourishment

- **Be alert to weight loss.** Most people lose weight toward the end of life, but weight loss also may signal other forces at work. If you see a precipitous weight loss, talk to your doctor to get an evaluation of your loved one's overall health.

- **Encourage your loved one to self-feed.** This little bit of independence and normalcy can make eating familiar again for the Alzheimer's patient. Often the person can still manage it with gentle direction. Put the food on a fork or spoon and put it into your loved one's hand. Guide it to her mouth if she does not do this. If your loved one can't use utensils, serve finger foods if you can. (See the tip below about swallowing.)

- **Watch for swallowing issues.** It's common for people with late-stage Alzheimer's disease to have difficulty swallowing, or to actually forget how to swallow. If this is the case, stay away from crunchy foods or those that require a lot of chewing. Serve soft foods, and thicken liquids like beverages and soups to prevent choking, and to keep the liquid from "going down the wrong way" and reaching the lungs. Thicker liquids are also easier to swallow. You can find food thickeners at your local pharmacy (or use cornstarch or unflavored gelatin).

- **Assist with feeding.** If your loved one needs assistance with eating, you will need to help. Use small bites, and make sure she chews and swallows before offering the next bite. Be sure to offer fluids between bites—your loved one may not recognize thirst, because this is one of the senses that diminish with Alzheimer's disease. If she refuses fluids, provide foods that have a high water content (like melon and sherbet).

- **Learn the Heimlich maneuver.** If your loved one struggles with swallowing, you need to be alert for the possibility of choking. Have her sit up straight with the head a little bit forward to minimize the possibility that she will choke. Check at the end of the meal to be sure no food remains in her mouth. Avoid foods that are hard to chew completely, like some raw vegetables and meats.

- **Switch to nonalcoholic beverages.** Maybe one of your father's favorite pastimes was having a few beers at the beach. There are alcohol-free beers and wines to help your loved one still feel social without the adverse effects of alcohol.

Sleeping and Sundowning

Problems sleeping are not uncommon in older adults, but they become more pronounced in people with Alzheimer's disease. To date, scientists do not really know how Alzheimer's disease causes sleep disturbances, but some specific issues develop that are most often found in people with Alzheimer's and related dementias.

- **Waking and staying awake during the night.** People with
  Alzheimer's may fall asleep fairly normally, but they do not stay
  asleep. They may get out of bed and wander around the house, or
  thrash around in the bed or call out for help. If you are a sole caregiver, you may find that your own sleep gets interrupted repeatedly
  during the night.

- **Shifts in the sleep cycle.** Many Alzheimer's patients doze off
  wherever they are sitting during daylight hours, napping for short
  intervals throughout the day. This makes it difficult for them to fall
  asleep or stay asleep at night. In fact, the Alzheimer's Association
  says that individuals in late-stage Alzheimer's spend as much as
  40 percent of the night in bed awake. As mentioned earlier, people
  with this disease flip day for night entirely, wandering during the
  night and sleeping through the day.

- **Sundowning.** About 20 percent of people with Alzheimer's disease
  become agitated in the late afternoon and early evening, right
  around sunset. This phenomenon can be very difficult for a caregiver to deal with, especially when it happens day after day.

One of the likely causes of sundown syndrome is a tiny area of the brain
called the suprachiasmatic nucleus, or SCN, which controls the circadian
rhythms that maintain a normal cycle of waking and sleeping. When
the SCN degenerates—as it does when a patient has dementia—the
onset of late afternoon and evening causes agitation, confusion, and
anxiety. It's easy for doctors to dismiss this disturbing behavioral
change as "just sundowning," but there's nothing trivial about it when
your loved one is upset.

In the shadows of late afternoon, people with Alzheimer's can become confused, anxious, and restless. They may pace or walk in a relentless route through the house, and they may talk about needing to be somewhere or find something in particular. In people whose symptoms include hallucinations and/or delusions, there may be an increase in their fears, suspicions, or visions, which can lead some people with this syndrome to become aggressive with their caregivers. It can be difficult for you to find a way to overcome these issues and calm the person; in fact, sundowning plays a significant role in caregiver burnout.

In addition to sundowning, some people with Alzheimer's also begin shadowing their caregivers—imitating their motions—in the late afternoon or early evening. You will find more information on this phenomenon in chapter 9.

Why does sundowning and shadowing occur? Science does not have a clear answer to this yet, though recent studies have provided new insight. A study at Ohio State University, published in 2011, found that mice of an advanced age with an Alzheimer's-like disease demonstrated increased levels of anxiety two or three hours before their sleep cycle would normally begin, just as humans with Alzheimer's disease do. These mice had an increase in an enzyme—acetylcholinesterase—before sleep, a chemical associated with anxiety and agitation in human beings. Drug therapies to slow or block this increase may come in the future, but none are available today.

Strategies to Aid Sleep and Reduce Sundowning

You can take some steps to reduce the effects of sleeplessness and sundowning, and observe their impact carefully to determine which of these things work for you.

- **Check for discomfort.** Your loved one may have an infection, pain, or other physical issue that causes her to wake up at night and become more agitated as the day goes on. Enlist your doctor's help to check for urinary tract infection, back pain, leg cramps, constipation, and other issues that can be remedied.

- **Keep your loved one busy.** Try to stave off daytime naps. Walks, hobbies, and activities that don't involve sitting in front of the television can prevent dozing.

- **Improve overnight comfort.** Perhaps your loved one would be more comfortable sleeping in a different bed or in a favorite recliner. A low-level light in the bedroom at night can help reduce the potential for confusion and panic when she wakes during the night.

- **Limit caffeine.** Coffee or tea served in the afternoon should be decaffeinated, and it may help to limit the amount of snacking the person with Alzheimer's does close to bedtime. Indigestion and acid reflux will wake people during the night.

- **Aromatherapy.** Essential oils have been reported as helping aid sleep and reduce stress. Your loved one, as well as you, can use aromatherapy in a diffuser, as oil on pressure points and feet, or in the bath. Jasmine, lavender, sandalwood, tangerine, and chamomile are just among the many options to try.

- **Remain calm.** Someone has to keep a cool, clear head in the face of increased anxiety. Your reassuring tone and serene expressions may help bring your loved one back to reality.

If night after night of sundowning and sleeplessness become too disruptive to you and your family, it may be time to look into an alternative living situation for your loved one. You'll find information about the options in chapter 11.

Toileting

As Alzheimer's disease progresses, bladder and bowel control becomes more of an issue. Many factors may be at play: The person may no longer recognize the urge to go to the bathroom, or she may know the urge but forget what to do once she gets into the bathroom. There may be an additional issue involved like a bladder infection, but once your doctor has ruled out any physical cause, it's time to accept the fact that this situation has arrived and determine the best way to deal with it.

No one wants to depend on another person to use the bathroom and clean up afterward, and it's a rare person who is willing to assist with this very personal, private function. If you are uncomfortable approaching this part of the caregiver role, don't beat yourself up. It's perfectly understandable that you find this task embarrassing or awkward. Your loved one probably is no happier about it than you, both because of the loss of privacy and because of what it signals: the approaching end of life.

....

Do not withhold fluids. Not only will this not solve the incontinence issue, but it could lead to dehydration, a dangerous condition that can lead to urinary tract infection, further incontinence, and increased confusion.

....

Toileting may be the crossroads point for you, the task that makes you decide it's time to look at assisted-living or skilled nursing care for your loved one. Trained professionals in home-care and senior community-based eldercare can help.

If you have determined that you would prefer to keep your loved one with you, then you will need to address the bathroom issue.

Your first impulse may be to reduce the amount of liquids the person with Alzheimer's consumes. *Do not withhold fluids.* Not only will this not solve the incontinence issue, but it could lead to dehydration, a dangerous condition that can lead to urinary tract infection, further incontinence, and increased confusion. Instead, provide at least six glasses of liquid daily—and as many as eight. This will stimulate the bladder to work properly, which will allow you to schedule trips to the bathroom. (Cranberry juice is particularly good for the bladder and urinary tract.) Give the last drink of the day at least two hours before bedtime, to minimize trips to the bathroom in the middle of the night.

Avoid caffeinated drinks: tea, coffee, cola, and other carbonated beverages and energy drinks. Not only do these stimulate the person with Alzheimer's, as discussed earlier in this chapter, but caffeine also has a diuretic effect that can increase incontinence. Instead, give herbal teas, decaffeinated coffee, fruit juice, seltzer or tonic water, and Jell-O.

A diet high in fiber can help with regulating bowels, allowing you to stick to your bathroom schedule. Whole-grain cereals and breads, fruits and vegetables, and fruit juice all can help you accomplish this. Fiber must be ingested with water to help ease elimination and avoid constipation.

Daily Strategies for Toileting

- **Use adult incontinence underwear.** Urination is a fact of life, so prepare for it by dressing your family member using these disposable garments. Change the wet garment as soon as you discover it—probably on his next trip to the bathroom.

- **Use waterproof bed pads.** Changing the bed every time there's an accident can leave you with no clean bedding when you need it—not to mention the wear and tear on your back. You and your loved one will be more comfortable if you take the precaution of using disposable bed pads that you can change in a moment.

- **Dress your loved one in clothes that are easy to remove.** This will save time and make the visit to the bathroom go smoothly. Adaptive clothing for people with dementia is available from a number of providers. See the Resources section of this book for more information.

- **Set a schedule.** To start, take your loved one to the bathroom for urination first thing in the morning, after each meal, and at bedtime. Set a schedule for a daily bowel movement as well by keeping track of approximately when this happens for several days. Learn to interpret the signs (fidgeting, anxiety, pacing, walking into the bathroom and back out again seconds later) that she may need to use the bathroom in between these times. People with Alzheimer's and other dementias cannot always ask to use the bathroom, or they may not want to bother you. Remember that asking is embarrassing to them.

- **Keep a log.** Make notes daily about when your family member uses the bathroom, and if her underwear is wet or dry when she goes. Soon you will see a pattern emerge, which will help you adjust the bathroom schedule to avoid as many wet visits as possible.

- **Prod gently.** Your loved one may not know what she is feeling when she has to go to the bathroom, so she won't tell you she needs to go or head for the bathroom herself. Ask quietly if she would like to go. Be discreet, especially if there are other people around, so as not to embarrass her.

- **Coach her along.** It may seem like the most instinctive and natural act there is, but for a person with Alzheimer's, toileting can be a complete mystery. Remind her of the steps involved as they come up. Ask her gently to move as you need her to so you can wipe and redress her, if she requires this kind of assistance. When she's finished, praise her. Never scold her if something goes wrong.

- **If something isn't right, call your doctor.** No bowel movement for several days is a medical issue that should be addressed by your loved one's physician. The same is true for urination, especially if there's a change in the number of times a day the patient goes. A bowel obstruction or dehydration is a serious condition that can be life threatening. At the very least, the pain and discomfort of such issues will exacerbate your loved one's confusion.

....

When you need to help your loved one with bathing, dressing, and toileting, it can be easy to slip into the language and tone you would use with a child. Your loved one is not a child, no matter how dependent on you she may have become. Think about how you would want to be spoken to if you were the person whose life had changed so dramatically. Treat your loved one with the same respect you did before she developed Alzheimer's.

....

Bathing

Alzheimer's disease can turn the basic acts of bathing and dressing into a frightening experience for the afflicted person. You can make this easier for both of you by making a plan and setting up the bathroom before bringing your family member in for a bath.

- **Timing is everything.** Choose a time of day when your loved one is at her calmest.

- **Be flexible.** Keep in mind that someone who always showered before she had Alzheimer's may now find the shower uncomfortable and scary. A bath may be a better bet.

- **Create a routine.** While the person with Alzheimer's may be unable to form memories of what you've done before, a routine will make it easier for you to keep track of what has been done and what needs to be.

- **Prep the space.** Have everything you will need handy, including the person's towels and robe.

- **Use a shower chair.** Place it in the right spot before your loved one steps into the shower or tub, so you don't need to reposition it with their full weight on it.

- **Narrate.** Tell the person what you are doing now, and what comes next. If she can assist, let her do as much as she can herself.

- **Use a shower wand.** A handheld showerhead in the shower or the bathtub will make rinsing off easier, faster, and safer.

- **Don't insist on a bath every day.** If your loved one gets little exercise and keeps clean, you may not need to do a complete bath every day. Try a sponge bath on alternate days.

Hygiene, Grooming, and Dressing

The process of getting dressed involves a wide range of skills and steps: choosing an outfit, taking off pajamas or other clothing, putting different clothes on, and using buttons, zippers, and other closures. All of these challenges can be too much for a person with Alzheimer's disease, especially in the later stages.

Perhaps your loved one once enjoyed a fashionable life with many wardrobe choices. Now that she has Alzheimer's disease, all of these clothes cause confusion and anxiety. Too many choices can lead to agitation, outbursts and accusations, or insistence that a long-lost wardrobe essential "must be here somewhere."

You can reduce the possibility of anxiety by minimizing the number of choices and by preparing the day's wardrobe.

- **Follow a schedule.** Getting dressed at the same time every day will help make the experience predictable.

- **Make choosing simple.** Set out two outfits and allow your loved one to choose between them. Keep all of the other clothing in a different room to reduce confusion.

- **Set up the clothing.** Once your loved one has chosen the day's wardrobe, place it in front of her in the order in which she will wear it. Hand her one piece at a time. This may make it possible for her to do most of the job on her own.

- **Modify the closures.** In a world of hook and loop fasteners such as Velcro, there's no need for your loved one to struggle with buttons and zippers. Choose clothing with hook and loop or snap closures, or replace buttons and zippers in familiar clothing with these easy and convenient materials. Items that pull on with no closures, such as elastic-waist pants, can make the process much easier.

- **Choose washable, wrinkle-free clothing.** Your loved one will inevitably have accidents at the dinner table, in the bathroom, and out and about. Make your life as easy as you can by avoiding delicate fabrics and sticking with items you can toss into the washer, shake out, and put away when they come out of the dryer.

Personal grooming becomes harder over time for people with Alzheimer's as they forget how to do daily tasks like combing their hair or brushing their teeth. Mundane items like a hairbrush, razor, or toothbrush may become foreign objects.

The amount of assistance you need to provide will change as the disease progresses.

- Do these tasks at the same time every day to create a routine that feels natural and predictable to your loved one.

- As with bathing and dressing, encourage the person to do as much as possible on his or her own, and plan ample time in your daily schedule to allow for this task.

- Continue to use their favorite toiletries so scents and textures are familiar.

- If your loved one has visited a hairdresser once a week for most of her life, continue with this schedule for as long as it is feasible.

- Simpler grooming implements may be more familiar and less threatening. Use an emery board instead of a metal nail file and an electric razor rather than a manual one with a sharp blade.

- Demonstrate a grooming activity—like brushing your hair—and urge your loved one to do it with you.

- Allow your loved one to hold the grooming tool while you guide the person's hand in shaving or brushing teeth. (This is a technique that professional home-health aides call "bridging.")

- If you need to brush the person's teeth, use a long-handled toothbrush or an electric toothbrush to make the task easier for you. Talk to your loved one's dentist about the best way to clean the person's teeth.

- Medications for anxiety and depression often cause dry mouth, which promotes bacteria in the mouth and prevents dentures from affixing properly. If this is the case with your loved one, use a mouthwash and toothpaste for dry mouth (like Biotene).

- If your loved one's dentures are old, have a dentist check for proper fit. Use a denture fixative that can compensate for dry mouth.

- Have your loved one rinse her mouth with mouthwash after each meal. This will make brushing teeth and flossing less time-consuming later.

- Keep your loved one's fingernails and toenails trimmed and clean. Many older people develop nail fungus and other issues with their toenails. Find a podiatrist who will take care of routine foot maintenance—a service that is covered by Medicare in many cases.

....

Should a person with Alzheimer's get dentures? After a dentist pulls all of your loved one's remaining teeth, it will take months for the swelling to go down before new dentures can be fitted. In the meantime, your dentist can create temporary dentures that will fit over the swollen gums, but your loved one may need several new sets of these as the swelling recedes. If all of this seems like too much, talk to your doctor about modifying the person's diet with food that's easy to chew, so she can keep her own teeth even if they give her some discomfort.

....

CHAPTER NINE

Understanding Communication

One of the most frustrating aspects of Alzheimer's disease—both for you and for your loved one—is the loss of verbal communication skills. People with Alzheimer's slowly lose the ability to find the word they want to use, sustain a train of thought, and understand what is being said to them. This can make it very difficult to determine what the person is asking or telling you.

As difficult as this aspect of Alzheimer's can be, there are coping strategies that can help soothe tempers and make communication a little smoother between you and your loved one.

Talking About the Illness

First, try to achieve a comfort level with talking about your loved one's condition with her, as well as with other family members and friends.

Very often, families feel that they should not tell the patient that he has Alzheimer's disease. "What he doesn't know won't hurt him," a family member may say to you, followed by, "He won't know what you mean anyway."

Families often assume that the person will become depressed and overcome by hopelessness if they know that they have Alzheimer's disease. The fact is that the Alzheimer's patient does know that something has gone terribly wrong with her memory, and pretending that nothing has happened does not make that fact any easier to take. If your loved one suspects that she has this disease, she has already begun to grapple with the concept.

Patients have the right to know what's wrong with them. Bringing the news out in the open and talking about it as a family will empower your loved one to be part of the planning and decision-making process for future care. The person with Alzheimer's also may feel relief in finally understanding the reason for the changes she has perceived, many of which may be frightening to her.

....

Your loved one knows that something is wrong with her memory. She has a right to hear the doctor's diagnosis.

....

Finally, talking about the illness openly allows your family to come together and have meaningful conversations with the person with Alzheimer's, instead of pretending that nothing has changed. This means that your family can be involved in your loved one's care by making visits, providing respite for you, cooking favorite meals, and including the person with Alzheimer's in holidays and family events. Keeping the diagnosis a secret only isolates you and your loved one—and that's a path to caregiver burnout.

When you share the diagnosis with your family member, be ready to answer questions about the disease and its progression. Emphasize the positive: People live for many years with Alzheimer's, and there are medications that can improve both memory and quality of life. Most of all, let the patient know she is not alone. You and your family will be with her every step of the way.

Changes in Communication

As the disease progresses, you will see your loved one's ability to communicate change. Exactly which of the challenges your family member will face depends on the stages of the disease (see chapter 7), but each individual case will progress in its own way.

- Your family member may substitute one word for another in an illogical way, leaving you to try to decipher what she might have meant.

- She may repeat the same word or question over and over, or make the same statement repeatedly in the space of a few minutes.

- Your loved one may describe a person or object instead of calling it by name.

- She may need additional time to compose her thoughts before responding to questions.

- She may string together syllables that do not form a word, perhaps in an attempt to approximate what she means.

- She will lose the thread of a conversation or the train of her thoughts, often in the middle of a sentence.

- If English was not her first language, your loved one may revert to speaking in her native language.

When you don't understand what she is saying, she may get angry, and you may eventually lose *your* temper. You may think any argument you have with your loved one will be forgotten in minutes, but you may continue to be angry long after the person has lost any memory of the interaction. There is no way to resolve the incident once your loved one has forgotten it happened, which can create anxiety, guilt, and frustration for you.

Verbal Outbursts

People with late-stage Alzheimer's may exclaim a word or phrase loudly and repeatedly, or they may yell for help if they misperceive a change in their environment. It's not uncommon for a person with Alzheimer's to cry out for the police if they don't recognize a person close to them, if they are being transported to an unfamiliar place (even if that place was familiar before the disease), or if they don't understand what they are expected to do.

Alzheimer's patients may demand to see a relative who has died, or may insist that it's time to go home when they are already at home. These declarations may have double meaning: The person may feel unsafe in her surroundings, which triggers long-term memories of a parent or of her childhood home. Check to see if the person feels pain, is hungry or thirsty, or is otherwise uncomfortable and in need of assistance.

Correcting the person or reminding your loved one that her mother has been dead for years won't be helpful. Despite prior knowledge of her mother's passing, your reminder may only trigger shock and renewed grieving, a situation you will have to deal with over and over. Instead, agree with the person and say something in acknowledgement of the demand. Follow this with redirection: "It would be nice to see her again, wouldn't it? Let's have something to eat."

By looking for the underlying emotion behind the verbal outburst, you can redirect your loved one and make her feel safer and more comfortable.

In late-stage Alzheimer's, the person may begin screaming or shouting a few words or syllables repeatedly, often with no discernible meaning. If this is the case, begin by looking to your doctor for a diagnosis. A number of conditions, including meningitis, traumatic brain injury, and toxicity—caused by liver or kidney disease—can cause symptoms including seemingly random screaming.

If there is no additional illness, the screams may be the only communication method your loved one can use to get something she needs. Determine if she is hungry, thirsty, in pain, or lonely. Relieving one of these conditions may put an end to the screams; if it works, make a note so you will remember for the next time.

Screaming can be troubling and difficult to tolerate. Try to remember that your loved one is not doing this to annoy or punish you; very often, she can't help this behavior. This is one more manifestation of Alzheimer's disease, and it will stop eventually as the disease progresses.

Repetitive Speech

How many times today has your loved one remarked, "Oh, you've changed your hair"? Repetitive statements are a classic symptom of Alzheimer's disease, one that can grate on a caregiver's nerves perhaps more than any other.

Remember, correcting the person or reminding them that you just answered the same question will not help; nor will ignoring the statement or question. Your family member does not remember asking it before, so she may be hurt or offended if you do not respond.

Try redirecting your loved one, focusing her attention on an activity or a different topic. If she is asking when an event will take place—such as the time dinner will be served—place a sign on the dining room table, such as, "Supper is at 6:00." The repeated question may be a demonstration of anxiety, so the visual reminder may take care of the issue.

If you are planning an event, don't tell your family member with Alzheimer's about it until just before it happens. The lack of anticipation will keep her from building up anxiety and asking you repeated questions about what will happen and when.

Shadowing

When your family member follows you around and mimics your behavior, or gets angry when you want some time to yourself, or you're busy in another room, she is shadowing—a common behavioral problem that affects people with Alzheimer's in the late afternoon and early evening. This may be accompanied by repetitive speech and interrupting you when you are speaking.

Determining the cause of this behavior can help you discourage it. Does it come at a particular time of day? What is going on in the house when this behavior begins? Is there anything that breaks the cycle and makes your loved one stop shadowing?

Giving your loved one a task of her own—folding laundry, sorting recyclables, stacking newspapers and magazines, or dusting—can help redirect her from shadowing to focus on her own project.

Get a lock for your bathroom door, so you can keep your loved one from following you in. Make sure it's a lock that can be unlocked from the outside, however, just in case your loved one goes in alone and locks the door.

Music or television can be a good distraction. Listening to music or an audiobook with headphones can help calm your loved one, and a favorite TV program may absorb her attention for a short time (as long as she is not inclined to have delusions about the people on the screen becoming real).

Ten Steps for Successful Communication

1. **Speak directly to the person with Alzheimer's.** Do not talk about her as if she is not in the room.

2. **Give the person plenty of time to respond to a question or to participate in a conversation.** Don't finish her sentences or interrupt her.

3. **Have conversations in a quiet place.** Turn off the TV or radio.

4. **Be patient.** Say, "There's no hurry, take your time."

5. **Look at the person when you speak to her and also when she responds to make it clear that you are listening and value what she has to say.**

6. **Ask one question at a time.** Don't give complex instructions.

7. **Ask closed-ended questions.** Yes or no answers can keep your loved one calm when searching for responses.

8. **Don't look for arguments.** If the person says something that sounds insulting or odd, keep in mind that the words she says may not be what she means.

9. **Use visual cues.** Touch or point to the thing you're talking about, to help your loved one make the link between the word and the object.

10. **Treat your loved one with respect.** Your family member is an adult who may have more understanding of your tone and facial expressions than your words. Baby talk is for babies, not for the person with Alzheimer's.

CHAPTER TEN

What Is Wandering?

Wandering and getting lost are often some of the earliest signs of Alzheimer's disease. Long before your loved one begins to repeat the same questions over and over or forgets the names of the grandchildren, she may lose her way home from work or the grocery store, or take a walk around the neighborhood and forget which way to turn to get back to the house.

Once Alzheimer's reveals itself more fully, wandering becomes a serious hazard. Understanding this particular symptom of the disease will help you predict potential wandering events and head them off before your loved one unwittingly puts herself in danger.

Why Does Wandering Occur?

Very often, wandering takes place when the person with Alzheimer's feels an urgent need to do something she once did daily, like go to work or go home to her family. With the distortion in her perception of reality that Alzheimer's can cause, she may not recall that she retired years ago or that she no longer lives in the home she shared with her parents.

Your loved one may open the door and walk out of the house, thinking she is going home to her childhood residence. If she is still driving—or if she has access to car keys—your loved one may take the car and drive away with the certainty that she has somewhere to go. In either case, she may suddenly realize that she has reached unfamiliar surroundings with no recollection of how she came to be there.

Some Alzheimer's patients decide to leave the house simply because they are bored or lonely and they want to find something interesting to do. Before long, however, once they have left their comfortable surroundings, they are likely to find themselves in a place they do not recognize.

Wandering Risk Factors

People with diminished mental capacity can face many dangers while they wander on their own in a neighborhood they do not recognize. They may lack the ability to ask strangers for help, making them unable to find a way back home. People they meet who do not understand the disease may treat them in ways that can be dangerous. At the very least, they may be exposed to bad weather without proper outer clothing. If they are missing for more than twenty-four hours, they may become dehydrated or weakened from hunger, or disoriented from lack of medication.

With all of these possibilities for accidents and injuries, many care-givers still believe that their loved ones will not wander, simply because they have not yet attempted to wander.

If the person is not found within twenty-four hours, the incidence of death or serious injury can be as high as 46 percent, depending on loca-tion and weather conditions.

How to Find a Missing Alzheimer's Patient

When you begin to suspect that your loved one is at risk for wandering, look into technologies that can help you prevent this from happening or assist you in looking for her if she does manage to leave the house.

An emergency medical-alert bracelet can be equipped with radio frequency identification (RFID), a system commonly used by law enforcement. If the person wanders and cannot be found, the RFID chip can be activated and used to help locate her. You can find such products by researching MedicAlert, the Alzheimer's Association's Safe Return,

LoJack Safety Net, and Emfinder. This may be a cost-effective solution, as the caregiver does not need to activate the device except in an emergency.

The Alzheimer's Association offers a tool called Comfort Zone, a Web-based location system that uses network-assisted GPS (A-GPS) to track the person both outdoors and indoors. Comfort Zone allows you to remotely monitor loved ones by receiving automated alerts when they have traveled beyond a preset zone. For a monthly fee, your loved one wears a locator device on a belt or wrist, and/or mounts one in the car if they are still driving. These devices communicate with the Comfort Zone application online, and you can access the information on the Comfort Zone Web site. If you can't access your Internet service, the association provides a 24-hour-a-day monitoring center that you can call for help in locating your loved one.

If your loved one wanders and you do not have any kind of tracking system in place to find her, a call to 911 may be your best recourse.

Ten Steps to Prevent Wandering

1. **Anticipate wandering.** With all of the other aspects of Alzheimer's disease to navigate, it's easy to forget that your loved one can wander off at a moment's notice without warning. Think of this symptom not as an "if," but as a "when."

2. **Listen for clues.** People with Alzheimer's may say, "It's time to go home," or "I have to go to work." This is a signal that they may take the initiative and walk out the front door.

3. **Redirect.** It won't help to say, "Mom, you are retired," because she is not likely to remember that fact. Instead, you might say, "But Mom, I need your help here in the house. Would you dust the living room?" Redirecting her to another useful activity may make her forget her urge to leave the house, while treating her need to do something meaningful with respect and dignity.

4. **Hang pictures on doors.** Wandering does not always include a far-off destination. Sometimes people with Alzheimer's forget where the bathroom is and try every door in the house, eventually letting

themselves outside and wandering off. Put a picture on each door in your house to help the person remember what's inside: a picture of a toilet on the bathroom door, one of a bed on the bedroom door, and so on.

5. **Hide the exits.** Buy a screen that looks like something else (a chest of drawers, for example) and install it on the inside of your door.

6. **Move the locks.** People with Alzheimer's may have no trouble opening a door or unlocking a conventional lock, as long as they can find it. Placing the deadbolt lock at knee level instead of shoulder level can make it invisible.

7. **Get some exercise.** A walk around the neighborhood with you or some light aerobics in front of the television may tire your loved one enough that she will not want to get up and leave.

8. **Provide meaningful activities.** Giving your family member something useful to do will redirect her interests. Helping you around the house can be enough to make her feel she has a purpose.

9. **Extend the illusion.** When your loved one says that she needs to go to work, respectfully tell her, "You're working from home today." Give her papers to sort, mail to read, or an old appliance to take apart—whatever may seem like work she did when she was employed. This type of redirection may not be effective for people in the early or moderate stages of dementia, but it can be very useful in keeping your loved one engaged if she has reached the later stages.

10. **Use technology.** If all else fails and you believe your loved one is at risk for wandering, choose a location management system that can help you pinpoint her location from your computer or smartphone.

Late-Stage Caregiving

CHAPTER ELEVEN

Alternative Care Options

No matter how good your intentions were at the outset of your time as a caregiver, a day comes when the job will become larger than one person can handle. The twenty-four-hour supervision, the disrupted sleep patterns, the need to transfer your loved one from bed to a chair and into and out of the bathtub, and the likelihood of wandering when your back is turned all might add up to more than you can possibly accomplish on your own.

Before you reach this point, it makes sense to build a plan for your family member's care that will be best for your loved one and for you. The eldercare industry provides many options that offer different levels of care, which are based on the needs of the patient—whether you want to keep your loved one at home with you or move her to a secure environment with other people who have similar needs.

How to Decide What's Best for You and Your Loved One

Once you determine that it's time to tap into outside resources, your first step will be to complete an official assessment of your family member's current state of health. This assessment is required by every home health care agency and eldercare community in the United States before they offer their services, to determine what level of care your loved one will require. The assessment also will determine what services Medicare will pay for if your family member requires home health care or a skilled nursing facility.

This assessment differs significantly from the process discussed in Chapter 1, which was geared toward diagnosing your loved one's dementia. The official assessment required by Medicare and eldercare communities involves a complete, comprehensive review of your family member's mental, physical, financial, and residential situation. The process of completing this assessment will reveal what activities of daily living your loved one cannot complete on her own, what hazards may exist in your living environment, what stage the disease has reached and what that means to your loved one's quality of life, and what kind of outside care you can afford. The result will be a plan that you can follow to meet current needs, determine what might be needed in the near future, and know what steps you need to take and how soon you need to act.

You can complete the assessment yourself, but you may want to bring in a qualified eldercare professional, such as a case manager or home health care professional, to do this for you. A case manager will not only help you gather the information for the assessment, but will guide you through the procedures of finding the right residential care—assisted living or a nursing home—when the time comes.

Your local chapter of the Alzheimer's Association, your community's Office of Aging, your doctor, a local hospital, or one of the organizations near you that offers information and guidance for caregivers of elderly people can provide contact information for case managers or home health-care professionals who handle geriatric assessment. Many home health agencies also provide this service.

A thorough assessment will include the following elements:

- Known diagnoses of chronic diseases, including Alzheimer's disease

- Unusual weight gain or loss in the recent past

- Ability to use the bathroom; incontinence

- Steadiness when standing and balance issues

- Insomnia or persistent fatigue

- Edema (swelling) in legs and feet, or other problems walking
- Vision and hearing problems
- Dental issues, including dentures
- Pain issues
- Circulation problems
- A list of your loved one's doctors
- Diagnoses of depression, anxiety, or psychosis
- Progression of Alzheimer's disease
- Recent hospitalizations
- Mood swings and anger issues
- Wandering and shadowing
- Loneliness and difficulty in retaining friends
- Lack of interest in communicating, including reading and writing
- Despondency and lack of interest in life in general
- A list of medications—prescription and over-the-counter
- Any homeopathic medicine in use, including herbal supplements
- Ability to take medications as directed, and any reactions you have seen
- Special dietary needs and favorite foods
- Ability to bathe, dress, call for help in an emergency, go up and down stairs, prepare meals and eat them, do housework, and drive
- Ability to maintain personal hygiene, including oral care, nail care, showering, shaving, neat hair, and clean clothes
- Hobbies and interests
- Reading preferences, like audio books or large-print books, or use of a magnifier

- Favorite TV programs
- The kind of exercise your loved one enjoys
- Languages they speak, and favorite topics of conversation
- Religious/spiritual background
- Accomplishments and life experiences
- Favorite social activities

In addition to these issues, the assessment will take into account the caregiving environment and any safety issues relating to the patient's current condition.

- Neighborhood safety
- Safe passages: width of passageways and hallways; clutter in the passageways; throw rugs and other slipping hazards
- Safe bathroom: Use of handrails, a seat in the tub, nonslip surfaces
- Patient's ability to spot a scam or scam artist whether on the phone or in person
- Patient's knowledge of contact information for family members
- Ability to participate at a senior center or other day program
- Membership in groups and organizations

Finally, the assessment will include questions about your loved one's financial situation.

- Health insurance coverage
- Long-term care coverage
- VA benefits
- Total assets, including the value of the home she owns

- Legal documents, including trusts, living will, and durable power of attorney (more on these in chapter 12)

- The name of the person's family attorney

Once the assessment is completed, a path will emerge from all the questions to help you determine whether a move to an assisted-living, eldercare, or memory care facility is warranted, or if in-home care with professional assistance will be the best thing for your loved one and for you. A professional case manager will talk to you as well about your own physical and mental state to help you decide if the caregiving role has become more than you believed it would be, and if you are experiencing the depression and burnout that afflict such a large percentage of full-time family caregivers.

Know Your Options

You may be surprised to discover the number of options available to help you secure the most appropriate care for your loved one. Sorting through them and understanding the differences can be confusing, so here is a breakdown to help you.

In-Home Care

In-home care involves a visiting nurse service or home health agency that will supply the level of care for which your loved one qualifies. This may include a daily visit by a home health aide for personal care, including bathing, shaving, and dressing your family member. If the assessment states that your loved one needs assistance with feeding and other activities of daily living, the aide could be with you for a longer portion of the day to assist with whatever activities your loved one needs. If there are medical issues that need to be addressed—particularly if your family member has multiple illnesses, such as diabetes, chronic obstructive pulmonary disease, heart disease, or a number of other issues—then a registered nurse may be needed to visit on a daily or weekly basis as the situation requires, to check vital signs, administer medications, and provide other medical assistance. All of these services are billed by the hour. If your loved one has long-term care insurance, the insurance company will pay for home health care up to a threshold set when your loved one purchased the insurance. If there is a medical need for the in-home care, Medicare may pay for some of it.

Respite Care

Respite care provides you with a break to keep you replenished for your full-time caregiving role. It's easy to get into the mindset that when you accepted the caregiver role, you agreed to an all-day, every-day venture in which you would take sole responsibility for your loved one. This assumption not only isolates you and your loved one but also is unhealthy for you. You need a break, and respite care is the way to get it.

Respite care can take place in your home and can be used in addition to in-home care. Volunteers come to your house to stay with your loved one while you leave to run errands or take some time for yourself. It can involve an adult day program that takes place during working hours, where you can bring your loved one in the morning and pick her up at the end of the day. During the day, she will participate in activities, perform some light exercise, enjoy a hot lunch and snacks, and even make some friends or spend time with people she already knows.

Some senior living communities provide short-term stays for elderly people specifically to help you when you need emergency relief. These stays are rarely covered by insurance, but they can be a lifesaver when you need to keep your loved one safe at a time when you must leave town, have surgery, or otherwise see to your own care. These overnight stays can be more than worth the cost when you consider the peace of mind they can restore.

· ·

Assisted living is a safe, comfortable environment that allows your loved one a sense of independence while all of her personal care needs are being met.

· ·

Assisted Living

Assisted living involves moving your family member to a senior living community in which she will have an apartment of her own. As a resident, your loved one will have meals with the other residents in a communal dining room, and staff members will clean the apartment, do laundry, and assist with activities of daily living. Your loved one's room will be equipped with a button to push if she needs help, and she will wear a pendant or wristband with a button to push if she falls or needs assistance. Chances are that your loved one qualifies for residence in a memory care unit of the community, which means that the outer doors are equipped with locks and alarms to alert the staff if any of the residents attempt to wander. All activities of daily living are handled by staff as the resident requires their assistance, from cleaning the resident's room to helping with dressing, bathing, and toileting. Medical staff members include nurses who can monitor vital signs and manage the residents' medications and are trained to handle the complications of Alzheimer's disease, including toileting, feeding, and laundry.

In addition to all of these personal care services, most assisted living communities have activities on-site that residents can choose to participate in, from games and puzzles to watching movies and sports. Staff members take the time to encourage residents to participate, which enriches the experience of living in a community and guards against loneliness and boredom. Assisted living is a safe, comfortable environment that allows your loved one a sense of independence while all of her personal care needs are being met. This can be an excellent environment for someone who has moderate-stage Alzheimer's with no other major medical issues. What's the downside? Assisted living is not paid for by medical insurance, so unless your loved one has long-term care insurance, it can be very expensive.

....

Many of today's modern facilities work to provide person-centered care, with a homelike atmosphere in which residents can enjoy their favorite pastimes as they receive the medical and personal care they need.

....

Nursing Homes

Nursing homes—also known as skilled nursing facilities—care for seniors in the last stages of life. They provide long-term medical care services for people with serious health conditions that require considerable care. Most seniors consider a move to a nursing home "the last exit on the highway," however with proper care, people in nursing homes often live for several years after their arrival. Many of today's modern facilities work to provide person-centered care, with a homelike, less institutional atmosphere in which residents can enjoy their favorite pastimes as they receive the medical care they need. Ask if the facility you're considering follows the Eden Alternative, a philosophy that works to diminish the resident's feelings of loneliness, helplessness, and boredom through person-centered care.

Even if you choose an assisted-living situation for your loved one, she may eventually need to move to a nursing home as her health declines. To make this move as low-impact as possible, try to choose a senior living community that offers much of, if not the full, continuum of care—from independent living to assisted living and finally to nursing home care. Facilities like these have the same senior medical staff at all levels, so your family member will see the same doctor, and the staff will know your loved one's medical history and be able to create the most comfortable environment for her.

Hospice Care

Hospice care or comfort care—also called palliative care—in the last days of life can be a godsend for someone who is dying, as well as for a grieving family. Hospice centers provide the compassionate care your loved one needs for a terminal illness while accommodating lengthy visits by family members, even if you wish to stay at your loved one's bedside overnight in the final hours of life. Some hospice centers offer support services for the family as well, including counseling, spiritual care (in centers with a specific religious background), kitchens where you and your family can prepare hot meals, and even massages. Some accept patients only in the last few days of life, while others care for people who may have up to six months of their lives remaining. Many visiting nurse services also provide hospice care in your home instead of in a facility. Medicare and Medicaid (in all but five states as of this writing) pay for hospice care in your home or in an approved center, making this option both affordable and preferable to a hospital when the time comes.

....

Families—especially children of elderly parents—often wonder if they should deplete their own retirement savings to take care of Mom or Dad in a nursing home. In most situations, this is neither required nor expected. First, "spend down" all of your parent's assets—including selling her home, liquidating her investments, and selling off any other property of value. Use the proceeds from these sales to pay for her care. Once all of these assets are just about gone, the person with power of attorney can apply for Medicaid on your parent's behalf. Consult an attorney to help you through this complicated process.

....

Discuss the Options

The next phase in your loved one's care is a decision you may be able to make on your own, but it makes sense to involve your family in the process. It should not come as a surprise to the rest of your family that you are bringing in outside help or, especially, that you are moving your family member to a facility. This move can be one of the most emotionally charged decisions anyone can make about a parent, sibling, or spouse, and you deserve to have the support of your family when you do it.

At the same time that you are making this stressful and emotional decision, you must deal with the financial issue as well. There's no way around it: senior care is extraordinarily expensive, with fees due on a monthly basis. If you do not have the power of attorney for your loved one, the person who does must take on the responsibility of dealing with Medicare, Medicaid, long-term care insurance companies, health insurance companies, the Veterans Administration, and any other authority that will be involved in paying for some portion of your loved one's care.

In virtually all cases, the person afflicted with Alzheimer's has to pay the majority of the cost of long-term care.

Bring the family together as best you can (again, you may need to use your favorite video chat app for those who are far away) to talk through the options and the financial means your loved one has available to pay for them. Share all of the information you have about the assessment, the long-term care options available, and the cost. When you make the decision as a family, you will have everyone's understanding of your loved one's situation, and fewer obstacles as you take the next steps.

How to Find Good Care

You can look at Web sites, ask friends for referrals, and narrow down your selection of assisted-living options and nursing homes in your area, but nothing replaces the in-person visit to the facility.

Before you visit, make notes on what you are hoping to find. You may want some specific services for your loved one, but here are some guidelines to get you started.

1. **Accreditation.** The American Association of Homes and Services for the Aging accredits the best skilled-nursing facilities, as do the state and local branches of this organization. The AAHSA has a rigorous review process that includes on-site visits, so you can feel confident that this facility has passed a strenuous inspection and maintains high standards.

2. **Seven-day admissions.** The best facilities offer admissions well into the evening, and on Sundays. People who arrive on a Sunday still need medical care—so when you visit each site, ask if your loved one can be seen by a qualified doctor and treated on a Sunday. If not, keep in mind that you may have to take your loved one to a hospital on a Sunday if the need arises.

3. **Medical capabilities.** Too many nursing homes have to turn away patients who need medical procedures or assistance. Something as simple as a medication delivered intravenously can send a resident

to the hospital. Make sure the facility you choose can handle these situations on-site.

4. **Staff gerontologists.** It's important that at least one doctor on staff is a specialist in gerontology—the area of science that pertains to aging. Your loved one may be on multiple medications and have a range of issues related to her Alzheimer's disease as well as her age, and a qualified gerontologist will take charge of the situation and sort it out to your family member's benefit.

5. **In-house pharmacy.** Your loved one should not have to wait hours for a taxi to bring a prescription from outside the facility. The best-skilled nursing situations have in-house pharmacies that can fill a prescription a few minutes after the doctor orders it. If the facility has no pharmacy, you may need to make the pharmacy run at a moment's notice.

6. **People in common areas.** When you walk through the skilled-nursing building, are all of the residents lying in beds in their rooms—or are they dressed and out in the common areas, socializing and sharing projects or puzzles? Quality of life does not end with admittance to a nursing home. Look for alert, active residents who are engaged with staff members or one another.

7. **Cleanliness.** It may seem obvious that a nursing home should be clean, but not all facilities have the same standards you may have for your loved one's surroundings. Take a good look around and see what the common areas and dining room look like. Use your nose as well as your eyes. Does the place smell like hospital disinfectant, or is there a pleasant smell you'd want to inhale every day?

8. **Pleasant, respectful staff members.** Do the staff members look like they want to work there? Are they whispering amongst themselves, or are they interacting with residents? Do they treat residents gently and with kindness? What you see among staff members may give you the best clues about how this facility runs.

9. **Person-centered care.** Moving to a skilled nursing facility does not have to mean that life has ended. Person-centered care is a new

culture for senior living, being put into practice across the country in all care levels, offered through senior living communities where enlightened leadership understand the role happiness plays in good health. Look for a place where residents' lives are filled with choices, from the kinds of daily activities they may have enjoyed throughout their life to what's on the menus for dinner. Some facilities have resident rooms clustered in "households," with a common living and dining area for a small group of residents and private bedrooms, creating a homelike atmosphere.

If your loved one has lived in her own home during much of your caregiving relationship, the move to a nursing home may have come abruptly, with the advancement of her Alzheimer's disease. She may be unable to participate in the process of sorting through and dividing up her own possessions, and your family members may not recognize the personal value many items have to her. Try to involve your loved one in these decisions as much as possible before she enters the nursing home. This will help reduce the sense of loss she will experience when she makes the move.

Ten Steps for Making the Transition

Your loved one may be the one who is moving, but you will feel an enormous change in your home when she is no longer your twenty-four-hour responsibility. Many caregivers experience a range of emotions for some time after their family member has relocated to assisted living or a nursing home.

1. **Be aware that you may feel lost** in your own home if that is where you were providing care for your loved one. Make a point of planning a nice evening for yourself on your first night without your loved one in the house. A quiet dinner and a good movie may be just the thing, especially if you prepare something you would not have cooked while your family member was there.

2. **Be ready for feelings of guilt,** especially if your loved one reacted negatively when she arrived at her new home. It will be hard to believe at first that you are doing the best thing, but you will accept this over time.

3. **Make the new setting homelike** as much as possible for your loved one. Bring decorative items from your loved one's former home, such as a favorite chair.

4. **Bring familiar items.** If your loved one made things, collected things, or has favorite objects from her travels, be sure to put them in her new room.

5. **Family photos are a must.** Add photos of children, grandchildren, and other family members—including a deceased spouse if there has been one, as your loved one probably will recognize that person.

6. **Decorate the room for the holidays** to help create a sense of time and season.

7. **Prepare yourself for an initial negative reaction.** When your loved one makes negative comments about the new home—and you can count on this—do your best not to take them to heart and feel as if you've done a terrible thing. You know that you and your family made this decision together, and that it is the best thing for your loved one. Say to her, "I know this is a big step. What is hard for you today?" Let her talk, listen to all of it, and don't offer solutions unless you have some. Remember that returning her to your home is not an option that is in her best interest.

8. **Understand that your loved one may not have a clear idea of where she is.** Depending on the advancement of the Alzheimer's disease, some people with Alzheimer's may think they have joined a private club, while others decide they're in a vacation resort. Some think their new environment is their place of work, and they get busy trying to figure out what their job might be. You know it's a nursing home, and it may be a blessing if they do not.

9. **Find out if there's a support group for family members at this senior living community.** Make a point of attending, especially in the first week if there's a meeting.

10. **Give yourself time to recuperate.** You may be surprised at how exhausted you feel. If you have been the sole caregiver for a long time, you have powered through as best you could and done what was necessary, and now it is time to rest. You have the right to get your energy and strength back in your own time. Take the time you need; you are not obligated to visit your loved one every day. You may feel a sense of restlessness yourself or that something is missing, since your free time was so limited for so long. Now that you have time and privacy, it can be challenging to remember what to do with them. Begin slowly by reaching out to friends, inviting them over, or even making a weekly date for coffee or a movie. Taking up an old hobby can give you a sense that you are slowly reclaiming yourself.

CHAPTER TWELVE

Outline a Plan for the Future

No one likes to think about the end of life, least of all someone who is devoting his or her time to caring for a cherished loved one. The time will come, however, when you will need to assist in settling this loved one's financial and legal affairs. If you can prepare for that time while she is living—and perhaps while she can assist you—then you will make the process easier for yourself when the time comes. The worst time to have to search for documents or sort through legal issues is while you are grieving.

In this chapter you will find useful checklists, definitions, and guidance to help you locate documents, consult with attorneys and bankers, and clear the way to completing the necessary tasks that come with the end of life.

Organize Financial Matters

Finding all of your loved one's financial information can be a tricky task, especially if you need to do so without her help or permission.

First, determine where the financial records are in your loved one's home (or in yours, if they moved in with you). Chances are there is a file drawer, cabinet, or box somewhere with bank statements and other paper records. A fireproof safe in the house might contain stock certificates, savings bonds, or other valuable papers and records.

You may find financial records in the house that date back decades. Many older people become uncertain about what records, statements, and paid bills to keep and what is safe to throw away. Here are the rules, according to the government website USA.gov (www.usa.gov):

- **Bank statements:** Keep for one year, unless you need them to support tax filings

- **Credit card records:** Until the bill is paid

- **Home purchase and improvement records:** As long as you own the property

- **Insurance:** As long as you own the policy

- **Investment statements:** Shred monthly statements, and keep annual statements until you sell the investment

- **Investment certificates:** Until you cash or sell the item

- **Loan documents:** Until you sell or pay off the item

- **Real estate deeds:** As long as you own the property

- **Receipts for large purchases:** Until you sell or discard the item

- **Service contracts and warranties:** Until you sell or discard the item

- **Social Security card:** Forever

- **Social Security statements:** When you get your new statement, shred the old one

- **Tax records:** Seven years from the filing date

- **Vehicle titles:** Until you sell or dispose of the car

- **Will:** Until updated

If you find large numbers of very old files, take them to an office supply superstore (like Staples) that shreds personal documents by the pound. This is a much better use of your time than sitting over a household shredder and pushing the documents through two or three pages at a time. You may have to make several trips to the store with a box at a time, but you can drop off the box and take care of other errands.

If your loved one was particularly computer savvy before her illness, she may have received her bank and credit card statements by email or accessed them online. If this is the case, look for financial software such as Quicken on her hard drive. The accounts may be listed there and reconciled up to a date before Alzheimer's disease made her unable to keep these records.

Keep a list of the accounts you find. Check bank statements to see if there is more than one account on the statement, such as a checking and a savings account. Annuities, certificates of deposit (CDs), and other investments may be recorded on bank statements as well.

You may need to locate a number of accounts and documents and determine who has access to each of these funds. While your loved one is living, the one person who can access financial accounts is the one named as durable power of attorney by your loved one. In some or all cases, there may be a second name on a bank account—a spouse, a child, or the power of attorney as a joint account holder. There also may be a beneficiary (also listed as a POD, or "payable on death") named on a bank account. Keep an eye out for these, as this beneficiary status will supersede instructions in a will.

If your loved one owns a home and you'd like to get an idea of what it might be worth, look for the most recent property tax assessment among her papers. This will give you the assessed value, which is often less than the selling value of the house. Consult a local real estate agent with expertise in the house's neighborhood to get a sense of comparative values of similar homes.

When you have all of the financial documents in one place and you've found the most recent balances for each bank account and investment, you can take a full inventory of your loved one's assets. This will tell you how much money you have to work with as you consider moving your loved one to assisted living or a nursing home.

Manage Legal Issues

If you are lucky and your loved one was conscientious about organizing her legal affairs before she was afflicted with Alzheimer's disease, you will find a notarized, original document indicating durable power of attorney. This document is essentially the key to the kingdom, the most straightforward way to access bank accounts and investments to pay for your loved one's care.

The person who has power of attorney can transact business on behalf of your loved one. As the attorney-in-fact, this person can sell your loved one's car, move money out of investment accounts and into bank accounts, sign checks, and make health care decisions. While the process of getting the power of attorney document recorded by all the banks, investment companies, insurance companies, pension holders, and health care organizations can be time-consuming and labor intensive, it will streamline your family's ability to function on your loved one's behalf for the foreseeable future.

If there is no power of attorney document, it is too late to have one drawn up once your family member has been diagnosed with late-stage Alzheimer's disease. He can no longer be considered "of sound mind," so he cannot sign legal documents. You will need to have a representative for your loved one appointed by a court of law to be able to access his accounts. This is not an expedient process, so as soon as you know that you need to take this step, consult an attorney who specializes in elder-care law to get the ball rolling. (The one exception to this is for the spouse, so if you are the caregiver for your wife or husband, you may be able to step in as power of attorney through joint tenancy. Consult your attorney to do this properly.)

In addition to the power of attorney, look for these documents in your loved one's papers. If you need to apply for Medicaid or Veterans Administration benefits to pay for your loved one's care, you will need many of these documents.

- Health care proxy/living will
- Health and life insurance policies

- Long-term care insurance policy

- Mortgage papers

- House deed

- Car title

- Birth certificate

- Death certificate of deceased spouse, if applicable

- Divorce papers, if applicable

- Military discharge papers

- Driver's license

- Passport

- Will

- Revocable living trust, if there is one

- Trusts and investments

- Safe deposit box keys

- Funeral arrangements (if preplanned) and cemetery plot papers

Some of these papers may be kept in a safe deposit box at your loved one's bank. If you don't find everything you need in the house, check bank statements for an annual payment for a safe deposit box.

Missing papers like birth, death, marriage, or divorce certificates can be retrieved from the state in which the events took place. The Centers for Disease Control and Prevention website provides links to every state's Vital Records office at www.cdc.gov/nchs/w2w.htm. There are fees for ordering missing records, but this may be the best way to get them quickly. Alternately, check with other elderly relatives to see if they may have the documents you need.

End-of-Life Issues

If your loved one took a particularly enlightened view of the end of life, and if she had the wherewithal to share her ideas with you about her last days and what comes after, then you are a very fortunate individual indeed. The fact is that most people do not want to talk about end-of-life issues, even when the time is all but upon them.

If you did not have the conversation at any time before your loved one developed Alzheimer's disease, perhaps she put things in order with her attorney some time ago. Look for advance directives like a health-care proxy or a living will. At the very least, these documents will tell you if your family member wants medical treatment to be withdrawn or withheld, in the event treatment is the only thing sustaining life. Not only is an advance directive a blessing to your loved one, but it also is a kindness done to you, taking the onus off of you for making the final decision.

If your loved one did not provide an advance directive before the advancement of her disease, most states allow the family to make decisions about end-of-life care for their loved one. Check with your attorney so that you can be prepared to do what is necessary when the time comes. If you believe that conflict will arise if your family has to make the decision together, try to resolve these conflicts in advance so you're not dealing with them on the day you must make a critical decision.

Some states also have their own Do Not Resuscitate form (also known as a DNR) for patients in nursing homes who have terminal illnesses and would prefer to die without interventions when the time comes. If you are a spouse or have power of attorney, you may be asked to sign such a form when your loved one enters a nursing home. Whether you wish to do this is entirely up to you, and it does not have to be done immediately. As your loved one's condition deteriorates, you may determine that the DNR is appropriate.

The most enlightened individuals did their families a tremendous favor and preplanned their own funeral. Among their important papers, you will find a folder or envelope from a funeral home or cemetery with a contract and all of the details laid out for you. This preplanning locks in the cost of the funeral on the day the contract was signed, and your loved one paid for this over time. This foresight will save you thousands of dollars and will keep you and your family from making extravagant decisions out of grief and guilt when your loved one dies.

If the funeral or memorial service has not been planned in advance, there's no time like the present to go ahead and do this. If you will reach a point at which you will need Medicaid to pay for your loved one's nursing-home care, Medicaid will require you to take some of the last remaining funds and preplan the funeral, to be sure that your loved one's estate provides the funds for this final act. The sooner you take care of this, the sooner you and your family will have peace of mind.

Finally, be sure that you have your loved one's most recent will, or that an attorney has one on file. Determine if there are any codicils—documents that provide instructions beyond the will itself—and if there is a revocable living trust that lists even more detail and specifics about items and to whom they will go at the time of death. If the details in these documents conflict, the revocable living trust is the document that supersedes the others. Your loved one's attorney will be able to help you with probate or any contests to the will and trust if the time comes.

Appendix
Resources

SUPPORT GROUPS

Alzheimer's Association support group locator:
www.alz.org/apps/we_can_help/support_groups.asp

Daily Strength, an online forum for Alzheimer's disease caregivers:
www.dailystrength.org/c/Alzheimers-Disease/support-group

Care Crossroads, an Alzheimer's Foundation of America support site
for caregivers: http://carecrossroads.org/cms/index.php

Care Connection, weekly teleconferences for caregivers of loved ones
with Alzheimer's disease, through the Alzheimer's Foundation of
America: www.alzfdn.org/AFAServices/careconnection.html

Family Caregiver Alliance—The National Center on Caregiving:
www.caregiver.org

Leeza's Place—A Place for Caregivers: www.leezasplace.org

CareGiving.com—Helping You as You Help Family Members
and Friends: www.caregiving.com

ONLINE RESOURCES DEDICATED TO ALZHEIMER'S DISEASE

Alzheimers.gov, the U.S. government resource for Alzheimer's disease and related dementias: www.alzheimers.gov

Alzheimer's Association: www.alz.org

Alzheimer's Disease Education and Referral Center: www.nia.nih.gov/alzheimers

Mayo Clinic on Alzheimer's Disease: www.mayoclinic.com/health/alzheimers-disease/DS00161

RESOURCES FOR ALZHEIMER'S CAREGIVERS

Alzheimer's Association online tools for caregivers: www.alz.org/care/alzheimers-dementia-online-tools.asp

National Adult Day Services Association: www.nadsa.org

NIHSeniorHealth, basic health and wellness information for older adults from the National Institutes of Health: http://nihseniorhealth.gov

AgingCare.com, for people caring for elderly parents, and for caregivers to connect with other caregivers: www.agingcare.com

Elder Care Online, for those caring for parents and other elderly loved ones: www.ec-online.net

Family Caregiver Alliance, the National Center on Caregiving: www.caregiver.org

ALZConnect, the Alzheimer's Association online community: www.alzconnected.org

HelpGuide.org— Support for Alzheimer's and Dementia Caregivers: www.helpguide.org/elder/alzheimers_disease_dementia_support_caregiver.htm

AlzOnline, support for Alzheimer's caregivers:
http://alzonline.phhp.ufl.edu

Silvert's Adaptive Clothing for Alzheimer's:
www.silverts.com/alzheimers-clothing/

Buck & Buck Adaptive Clothing: www.buckandbuck.com

References

Agingcare.com. "How to Prevent Back Injuries When Lifting Someone." Accessed December 3, 2013, www.agingcare.com/Articles/ Practicing-Ergonomics-in-a-Home-Care- Environment-122277.htm

Allina Hospitals and Clinics. "Preventing Back Injuries Among Caregivers." Accessed December 3, 2013, www.mnhospitals.org/Portals/0/Documents/ ptsafety/lift/allina_SP_movement_annual_ed_(revised-11-25).pdf

Alzheimer's Association. "10 Early Signs and Symptoms of Alzheimer's," 2009. Accessed December 3, 2013, www.alz.org/alzheimers_disease_10_signs_of_alz- heimers.asp

Alzheimer's Association. "2013 Facts and Figures Fact Sheet." Accessed December 3, 2013, www.alz.org/documents_custom/2013_facts_figures_fact_ sheet.pdf

Alzheimer's Association. "Communication: Tips for Successful Communication at All Stages of the Disease." Accessed December 3, 2013, www.alz.org/national/ documents/brochure_communication.pdf

Alzheimer's Association. "Alternative Treatments." Accessed December 12, 2013. http://www.alz.org/alzheimers_disease_alternative_treatments.asp#Caprylic_ Acid.

Alzheimer's Association, New York City Chapter. "Incontinence and Toileting." Accessed December 3, 2013, www.alznyc.org/caregivers/incontinence.asp

Alzheimer's Association, New York City Chapter. "Sundowning and Shadowing." Accessed December 3, 2013, www.alznyc.org/caregivers/sundowning.asp

Alz.org Research Center. "Current Alzheimer's Treatments." Accessed December 3, 2013, www.alz.org/research/science/alzheimers_disease_treatments.asp#approved

AARP Foundation. "Prepare To Care: A Planning Guide for Families." Accessed December 3, 2013, http://assets.aarp.org/www.aarp.org_/articles/foundation/aa66r2_care.pdf

Bedrosian, Tracy A., Kamilya Herring, Zachary M. Weil, and Randy J. Nelson. "Altered Temporal Patterns of Anxiety in Aged and Amyloid Precursor Protein (APP) Transgenic Mice." *Proceedings of the National Academy of Sciences of the United States of America PNAS* (2011). Accessed December 3, 2013, doi: 10.1073/pnas.1103098108

Bixler, Jennifer. "More than 1 in 10 in U.S. Take Antidepressants," 2011. Accessed December 3, 2013, http://thechart.blogs.cnn.com/2011/10/19/more-than-1-in-10-in-u-s-take-antidepressants/

CareConversations.org. "Helping Your Loved One Transition to Skilled Nursing Care." Accessed December 3, 2013, http://careconversations.org/Planning_Preparing/Helping_With_The_Transition.aspx

"Caregiver Stress & Burnout: Tips for Recharging and Finding Balance." Accessed December 3, 2013, www.helpguide.org/elder/caregiver_stress_burnout.htm

Center on Aging Society. "How Do Family Caregivers Fare? A Closer Look at Their Experiences," Data Profile, Number 3. Washington, DC: Georgetown University, 2005. Accessed December 3, 2013, http://ihcrp.georgetown.edu/agingsociety/pdfs/CAREGIVERS3.pdf

Cohen, Elizabeth. "How to Limit Alzheimer's Wandering." Last updated November 10, 2011. Accessed December 3, 2013, www.cnn.com/2011/11/10/health/alzheimers-lost-empowered-patient/

Dr. Vicki. "Eight Tips to Managing Caregiver Guilt." Today's Caregiver. Accessed December 3, 2013, www.caregiver.com/articles/caregiver/managing_caregiver_guilt.htm

Eden Alternative. "Our 10 Principles." Accessed December 3, 2013, www.edenalt .org/our-10-principles

Help for Alzheimer's Families, Home Instead Senior Care. "How Do I Talk to Dad About His Diagnosis?" Accessed December 3, 2013, www. helpforalzheimersfamilies.com/alzheimers-dementia-dealing/guide/ sharing-alzheimers-diagnosis/

Hill, Carrie, Ph.D. "Caregiver Transitions: How Caregiving Changes Over Time." Last updated January 7, 2009. Accessed December 3, 2013, http://alzheimers .about.com/od/caregiving/qt/transitions.htm

Illinois Council on Long Term Care. "Understanding the Transition to Life in a Nursing Home." Accessed December 12, 2013. http://nursinghome.org/fam/ fam_004.html.

Kallmyer, Beth, and Nancy Cullen. "Aging Safely at Home: The Use of Technology to Address Location Management and Wandering for Persons with Alzheimer's Disease." Accessed December 3, 2013, www.caremanager.org/wp-content/ uploads/Technology_Aging_Safely_at_Home.pdf

Kennard, Christine. "Alzheimer's Caregiver Tips: Coping with Screaming and Other Loud Repetitive Vocalizations," 2011. Accessed December 3, 2013, www. healthcentral.com/alzheimers/c/57548/142043/vocalizations/

Kennard, Christine. "Caregiver Tips on Managing Confusion in Alzheimer's Disease," 2009. Accessed December 3, 2013, www.healthcentral.com/ alzheimers/c/57548/78464/caregiver-tips/

Khachiyants, Nina, David Trinkle, Sang Joon Son, and Kye Y. Kim. "Sundown Syndrome in Persons with Dementia: An Update." *Psychiatry Investigation* 8, no. 4 (December 2011): 275–87. doi:10.4306/pi.2011.8.4.275.

Lake Region State College for the North Dakota Department of Human Services, Aging Services Division. "Training for Caregivers of Individuals With Dementia," 2006. Accessed December 3, 2013, www.nd.gov/dhs/info/pubs/docs/2006-aging-alzheimer-training-manual-for-caregivers.pdf

Lee, V. M., T. W. Wong, and C. C. Lau. "Home Accidents in Elderly Patients Presenting to an Emergency Department." *Accident and Emergency Nursing* 7, no. 2 (April 1999): 96–102. http://www.ncbi.nlm.nih.gov/pubmed/10578721.

Mayo Clinic. "Alzheimer's: Tips for Effective Communication." Accessed
   December 3, 2013, www.mayoclinic.com/health/alzheimers/AZ00004/

Mersky Leder, Jane. "Adult Sibling Rivalry." *Psychology Today*. Last modified
   June 20, 2013. http://www.psychologytoday.com/articles/199301/adult-
   sibling-rivalry.

National Institute on Aging, National Institutes of Health. "Caregiver Guide: Tips
   for Caregivers of People with Alzheimer's Disease." Accessed December 3, 2013,
   www.nia.nih.gov/sites/default/files/alzheimers_caregiver_guide.pdf

National Institute on Aging, National Institutes of Health. "Home Safety for People
   with Alzheimer's Disease." Accessed December 3, 2013, www.nia.nih.gov/sites/
   default/files/home_safety_for_people_with_alzheimers_disease_0.pdf

National Sleep Foundation. "How Much Sleep Do We Really Need?" Accessed
   December 3, 2013, www.sleepfoundation.org/article/how-sleep-works/
   how-much-sleep-do-we-really-need

Purcell, Maud, LCSW. "Guilt: The Crippling Emotion." PsychCentral.com.
   Accessed December 3, 2013, http://psychcentral.com/lib/guilt-the-crippling-
   emotion/000722

Reinhard, Susan C., Barbara Given, Nirvana Huhtala Petlick, and Ann Bemis.
   "Supporting Family Caregivers in Providing Care." *Patient Safety and Quality:
   An Evidence-Based Handbook for Nurses*. Rockville, MD: AHRQ Publishing,
   2008. Accessed December 3, 2013, www.ncbi.nlm.nih.gov/books/NBK2665/

Rubinstein, Nataly. "5 Frustrating Behaviors of Alzheimer's Patients ... and How to
   Handle Them." *Health News Digest*, October 6, 2011. www.healthnewsdigest
   .com/news/Alzheimer_Issues_680/5_Frustrating_Behaviors_of_Alzheimer_s_
   Patients_and_How_to_Handle_Them_printer.shtml

Samaha, Gail M. "Family Caregiver: Making Your Job Easier." Accessed
   December 3, 2013, www.agingcare.com/Articles/caregiving-make-
   life-easier-137419.htm

Scott, Paula Spencer. "5 Tips for Smoother Social Visits for Someone With
   Dementia." Accessed December 3, 2013, www.caring.com/articles/smoother-
   social-visits-for-dementia

Scott, Paula Spencer. "How to Communicate Better with Someone Who Has Early-Stage Alzheimer's." Accessed December 3, 2013, www.caring.com/articles/how-to-communicate-with-alzheimers-patients

Spoonholz, Melanie. "Physical Therapy and Rehabilitation for Alzheimer's and Dementia." Accessed December 3, 2013, www.agingcare.com/Articles/physical-speech-therapy-alzheimers-dementia-143469.htm

Tartakovsky, Margarita, MS. "5 Strategies for Self-Compassion." Accessed December 3, 2013, http://psychcentral.com/blog/archives/2012/06/27/5-strategies-for-self-compassion/

University of Pittsburgh Medical Center (UPMC.com). "Thickened Liquids: Nectar-Thick." Accessed December 3, 2013, www.upmc.com/patients-visitors/education/nutrition/pages/thickened-liquids-nectar-thick.aspx

USA.gov. "Managing Household Records." www.usa.gov/Topics/Money/Personal-Finance/Managing-Household-Records.shtml

U.S. Department of Health and Human Services. "Health Information Privacy." www.hhs.gov/ocr/privacy/

U.S. National Library of Medicine and National Institutes of Health. "Aging Changes in the Bones – Muscles – Joints." Accessed December 3, 2013, www.nlm.nih.gov/medlineplus/ency/article/004015.htm

WebMD: Alzheimer's Disease Health Center. "Sundowning." Accessed December 3, 2013, www.webmd.com/alzheimers/guide/sundowning-causes-symptoms-treatments

Zarit, S. "Assessment of Family Caregivers: A Research Perspective." In "Family Caregiver Alliance (Eds.), Caregiver Assessment: Voices and Views from the Field," report from a National Consensus Development Conference, San Francisco: Family Caregiver Alliance, April 2006.

Zieve, David, David R. Eltz, Stephanie Slon, and Nissi Wang, eds. "Aging Changes in the Senses." With contribution by David C. Dugdale. MedlinePlus. Last modified November 10, 2012. http://www.nlm.nih.gov/medlineplus/ency/article/004013.htm.

Index